Contents

KT-528-926

Foreword

Carol L. Cox
PhD, MSc, MA Ed., PG Dip Ed, BSc (Hons), RN
Professor of Nursing, Advanced Clinical Practice
City University, London

Practice is advancing, and the future holds a time of dynamic change and challenge in stoma care nursing. Today's nurses can look forward to an opportunity to broaden their ability to advocate for the needs of patients with stomas. Porrett and McGrath's book is a journey in practice that will help nurses develop basic skills in stoma care and also broaden their expertise upon which professional nursing is built. This book provides an impressive approach to the provision of quality care. It lays the foundations of practice that nurses should strive to achieve so that patients with stomas receive appropriate care that meets their specialised needs.

Throughout this book nurses are shown how to develop and refine their ability to apply more advanced practice and analytical thinking to clinical situations. The authors and contributors have endeavoured to respond to the ever-changing nature of specialised stoma care nursing by incorporating the most up to date, evidence-based and clinically relevant information available. Thus each chapter provides nurses with a clear perception of the many complex and inter-related principles that need to be followed to achieve excellence in stoma care nursing practice.

It is apparent that considerable thought has been given to the nurse as a learner when introducing the complex issues associated with stoma care nursing. Each chapter provides the nurse with a clear set of the learning objectives that will be addressed as well as what the nurse should be able to achieve at the conclusion of the chapter.

Approaches to support patients including physical and psychological interventions that reduce suffering, speed recovery and enhance knowledge about how the patient can be taught to self-care for a stoma. After reading this book nurses can be assured that they will have advanced their practice knowledge and skills so that the care they provide is appropriately prioritised and built around the needs of the patient.

This book makes an important contribution to preparing nurses to become effective practitioners within the field of stoma care. It is written by an impressive team of contributors who are considered experts in the field. They bring a wealth of experience in caring for patients with stomas into the development of this book that will aid all nurses embarking on or advancing their career in stoma care nursing with the knowledge they need to remain up to date with contemporary stoma care nursing practice.

Preface

Stoma care nursing developed as a specialism in the UK after the first course in 1972 and the inception of the first stoma care nursing post at St Bartholomew's Hospital, London. The role of the stoma care nurse specialist (SCN) is wide ranging and includes pre-operative support, postoperative teaching and follow-up in the community. Despite the key role of the SCN in the support and clinical management of the patient with a stoma, the ward nurse has a large part to play in the patient's rehabilitation and care.

We have attempted to deal with all aspects of stoma care but have focused particularly on those areas which the ward nurse will commonly see and be involved in. Patients with a stoma often feel stigmatised by the nature of their condition and many find the subject embarrassing and difficult to discuss. It is often the informed and empathic ward nurse who supports, educates and advises patients with a stoma throughout their treatment pathway, and the positive impact these nurses can have on the quality of care the patient receives should not be underestimated. Equally, an uninformed nurse may significantly hinder a patient's psychological adaptation to their altered body image by a simple non-verbal signal.

We hope that the reader will find the information contained in this text useful in the management and understanding of patients with a stoma and that it supports clinical practice at a ward level.

Anthony McGrath and Theresa Porrett

Contributors

Patricia Black
(contributor to
Chapter 4)

MSc, SRN, RCNT, FPA Cert, FETC, DipN,
ENB 980, Adv. Stoma Care Cert.
Senior Clinical Nurse Specialist
Stoma/Colorectal
Course Leader of 'Foundations in Stoma Care',
in association with Buckingham Chilterns
University College
Colorectal Department
The Hillingdon Hospital NHS Trust
Middlesex

Jude Cottam
(contributor to
Chapter 6)

FAETC, RGN, Msc
Clinical Nurse Specialist (Stoma and Colorectal)
Colorectal Nursing Service
Bedford Hospital
Bedford

Juliette Fulham
(contributor to
Chapter 11)

RGN, ENB 998, Dip. Oncology Nursing
Stoma Care Nurse
Colorectal Department
The Hillingdon Hospital NHS Trust
Middlesex

Antoinette Johnson
(contributor to
Chapters 7 & 9)

RGN, Diploma in Nursing
Clinical Nurse Specialist Stoma Care
Homerton University Hospital NHS Trust
Homerton Row
London

Julia Williams
(contributor to
Chapter 12)

RGN, MEd., BSc (Hons), Dip. D/N
Lecturer in Gastrointestinal Nursing
St Bartholomew School of Nursing
City University
London

Anatomy and Physiology of the Bowel and Urinary Systems

1

Anthony McGrath

INTRODUCTION

The aim of this chapter is to increase the reader's understanding of the small and large bowel and urinary system as this will enhance their knowledge base and allow them to apply this knowledge when caring for patients who are to undergo stoma formation.

LEARNING OBJECTIVES

By the end of this chapter the reader will have:

❏ an understanding of the anatomy and physiology of the small and large bowel;
❏ an understanding of the anatomy and physiology of the urinary system.

GASTROINTESTINAL TRACT

The gastrointestinal (GI) tract (Fig. 1.1) consists of the mouth, pharynx, oesophagus, stomach, duodenum, jejunum, small and large intestines, rectum and anal canal. It is a muscular tube, approximately 9 m in length, and it is controlled by the autonomic nervous system. However, while giving a brief outline of the whole system and its makeup, this chapter will focus on the anatomy and physiology of the small and large bowel and the urinary system.

The GI tract is responsible for the breakdown, digestion and absorption of food, and the removal of solid waste in the form of faeces from the body. As food is eaten, it passes through each section of the GI tract and is subjected to the action of various

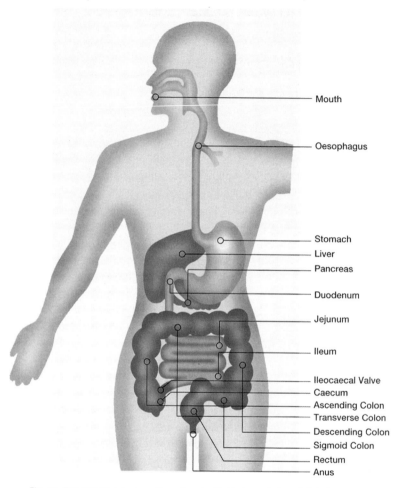

Fig. 1.1 The digestive system. Reproduced with kind permission of Coloplast Ltd from *An Introduction to Stoma Care* 2000

digestive fluids and enzymes (Lehne 1998). The salivary glands switch into action as soon as food enters the mouth, and as the food continues on its journey, enzymes found in the stomach, small intestine, the pancreas and the liver continue the process. It is this secretion of fluids that helps maintain the function of the tract (Tortora & Grabowski 2001).

Lining of the GI tract

Throughout the GI tract, the walls are made up of mucous membrane, constructed in such a way that the various parts can act independently of each other. The walls of the GI tract consist of four layers. These are the:

- adventitia;
- muscularis;
- submucosa;
- mucosa.

Adventitia

The adventitia or outer layer consists of a serous membrane composed of connective tissue and epithelium. In the abdomen it is called the visceral peritoneum. It forms a part of the peritoneum, which is the largest serous membrane of the body (Thibodeau & Patton 2002).

Peritoneum

The peritoneum is the serous membrane that lines the abdominal and pelvic cavities, and covers most abdominal viscera. It is a large closed sac of thin membrane which has two layers:

- the parietal peritoneum, which lines the abdominal and pelvic cavities;
- the visceral peritoneum which covers the external surfaces of most abdominal organs, including the intestinal tract.

The serous membrane is made up of simple squamous epithelium and a supporting layer of connective tissue. The potential space between the visceral and parietal layers is known as the peritoneal cavity and contains serous fluid. In some diseases, such as liver disease, the peritoneal cavity can fill up with serous fluid called ascites. Some organs protrude into the abdominal cavity but are not encased in the visceral peritoneum. The kidneys lie in this type of position and are said to be 'retroperitoneal'.

The folds of the peritoneum bind the organs to the cavity walls and to each other. The folds include the mesentery, the lesser omentum, the greater omentum and the faciform ligament. These folds contain the nerve, blood and lymph supply to the abdominal organs. The mesentery is attached to the posterior abdominal wall and this binds the small intestine to the abdominal wall. The lesser omentum arises from the lesser curvature of the stomach and extends to the liver. The greater omentum is given off from the greater curvature of the stomach, forms a large sheet that lies over the intestines, and then converges into parietal peritoneum. The falciform ligament attaches the liver to the anterior abdominal wall and to the diaphragm (Ross *et al.* 2001).

Muscularis

The muscularis mostly consists of two layers of smooth muscle, which contract in a wave-like motion. The exceptions can be found in the mouth, pharynx and the upper oesophagus, which are made of skeletal muscle that aids swallowing. The two smooth muscle layers consist of longitudinal fibres in the outer layer and circular fibres in the inner layer. The contraction of these two layers of muscle assists in breaking down the food, mixing it with the digestive secretions and propelling it forward. This action is referred to as peristalsis. Peristaltic action looks like an ocean wave moving through the muscle. The muscle constricts and then propels the narrowed portion slowly down the length of the organ forcing anything in front of the narrowing to move forward.

Between the two muscle layers the blood vessels, lymph vessels and the major nerve supply to the GI tract can be found. The nerve supply is called the mesenteric or Auerbach's plexus, and it consists of both sympathetic and parasympathetic nerves. It is mostly responsible for GI motility, which is the ability of the GI tract to move spontaneously (Tucker 2002; Martini 2004).

Submucosa

The submucous layer is highly vascular as it houses plexuses of blood vessels, nerves and lymph vessels, and tissue. It consists of connective tissue and elastic fibres. It also contains the submucosal or Meissner's plexus, which is important in controlling the secretions in the GI tract (Martini 2004).

Mucosa

The mucosa is a layer of mucous membrane that forms the inner lining of the GI tract. It is made up of three layers:

- a lining layer of epithelium, which acts as a protective layer in the mouth and oesophagus, and has secretory and absorptive functions throughout the rest of the tract;
- the lamina propria, which supports the epithelium by binding it to the muscularis mucosae and is made up of loose connective tissue that contains blood and lymph vessels;
- the muscularis mucosae layer, which contains smooth muscle fibres (Siegfried 2002).

SMALL INTESTINE

The small intestine begins at the pyloric sphincter and coils its way through the central and lower aspects of the abdominal cavity and joins the large intestine (colon) at the ileocaecal valve. The small intestine is divided into three separate segments: the duodenum, jejunum and ileum. The nerve supply for the small bowel is both sympathetic and parasympathetic.

It is approximately 6.5 m long and has a diameter of approximately 2.5 cm. The walls of the small intestine consist of the same four layers as the rest of the GI tract, however, both the mucosal and submucosal layers are modified. The mucosal layer consists of many glands called intestinal glands. These glands are lined with glandular epithelium, and they secrete intestinal juice. The submucosa in the duodenum contains glands that secrete mucus which is alkaline, this is designed to protect the small intestine walls from the acid in chyme and prevent the enzymes from acting on the walls. The small intestine is further modified in that throughout its length the epithelium covering the lining and the mucosa is made up of simple columnar epithelium. This contains both absorptive and goblet cells. If you were to examine the small intestine using a powerful microscope you would note that the absorptive cells actually contain projections described as 'finger-like'. The projections are known as microvilli and allow the small intestine to deal with larger amounts of digested nutrients, having simply increased the surface area for digestion (Thibodeau & Patton 2002; Ellis 2004).

The mucosa has a velvety appearance because its surface is made up by a series of villi. There are approximately 20–40 villi per square millimetre and these also increase the absorptive and digestive surface of the small intestine. They are about 0.5–1 mm long and their walls are made up of columnar epithelial cells with tiny microvilli. The cells enclose a network of blood and lymphatic capillaries. The lymphatic vessels are known as lacteals. Nutrients pass via the blood capillaries and lacteals into the cardiovascular and lymphatic systems (Tortora & Grabowski 2002).

The surface area of the small intestine is further increased by the presence of circular folds about 10 mm high. These are unlike the rugae in the stomach that flatten out, in that they remain in place. They cause the chyme to twist around as it moves through the small intestine. This assists the digestive and absorptive processes. Throughout the mucous membrane in the small intestine numerous lymph nodes occur at irregular intervals. The nodes are known as either solitary or aggregated lymphatic follicles (Peyer's patches) that occur in groups, and they are found mostly in the ileum (Watson 2000; Ross *et al*. 2001).

Thus, the main function of the small intestine is digestion and absorption and its makeup is designed to help this process. The chyme is broken into small molecules that can be transported across the epithelium and into the blood stream. This occurs in the presence of pancreatic enzymes and bile, which are important in the digestive process. The small intestine absorbs most of the water, electrolytes (sodium, chloride, potassium) and glucose (amino acids and fatty acid) from the chyme. The small intestine not only provides nutrients to the body but also plays a critical role in water and acid–base balance (Tortora & Grabowski 2002; Martini 2004).

The chyme from the stomach moves along the small intestine at approximately 1 cm/min. As the small intestine is about 6.4 m in length, chyme can remain in the small intestine for up to eight hours. The chyme is moved along by peristaltic movements, which are controlled by the autonomic nervous system. Digestion is completed in the small intestine with the aid of juices from the liver and pancreas. Waste is then transported to the large intestine for disposal.

The superior mesenteric artery supplies the whole of the small intestine and venous blood is drained by the superior mesenteric vein that links with other veins to form the hepatic portal vein (Watson 2000; Ross *et al*. 2001).

Duodenum

This is approximately 25 cm in length and it curves around the head of the pancreas. In the mid-section of the duodenum there is an opening from both the pancreas and the common bile duct. This opening is controlled by the sphincter of Oddi.

Jejunum
This is approximately 2.5 m in length and extends to the ileum.

Ileum
This is the terminal part of the small intestine that ends at the ileocaecal valve. It measures about 3.5 m in length. The ileum will usually empty approximately 1.5 litres of fluid into the colon each day.

Pancreas
The pancreas is attached to the duodenum and lies posterior to the greater curvature of the stomach. When chyme enters the duodenum the hormone secretin is released and this stimulates the pancreas to secrete its juices. The pancreatic juices pass through the pancreatic ducts into the duodenum to aid digestion by neutralising the acid to continue the digestive process (Ross *et al.* 2001).

Liver and gall bladder
The liver is situated in the right hypochondrium and extends into the epigastric region. Bile, which is produced in the liver, passes from the hepatic ducts into the cystic duct prior to entering the gall bladder for storage. When fatty foods are detected in the duodenum the hormone cholecystokinin is secreted. This causes the gall bladder to contract thus pushing the bile into the duodenum to emulsify the fatty food (Kumar & Clark 1998; Page 2001).

LARGE INTESTINE
The large intestine is so called because of its ability to distend. It forms a three-sided frame around the small intestine leaving its inferior area open to the pelvis. It is designed to absorb water from the contents of the small intestine that pass into it. Although the small intestine absorbs some water this process is intensified in the large intestine until the familiar semisolid consistency of faeces is achieved. The large intestine is

approximately 1.5 m in length and extends from the ileum to the anus. Its size decreases gradually from the caecum, where it is approximately 7 cm in diameter, to the sigmoid, where it is approximately 2.5 cm in diameter (Keshav 2003). The large intestine has four segments: the caecum, colon, rectum and anal canal. The colon is divided into four sections: the ascending colon, transverse colon, descending colon and sigmoid colon.

The large intestine also houses a variety of bacteria. These bacteria, known as commensals, live happily in the bowel and generally do not cause any problems. In fact, they play an important part in digestion – they ferment carbohydrates and release hydrogen, carbon dioxide and methane gas. The bacteria also synthesise a number of vitamins such as vitamin K and some B vitamins. They are also responsible for breaking down the bilirubin into urobilinogen, which gives the faeces its characteristic brown colour. However, outside the bowel the bacteria can cause illness and even death.

The blood supply to the large intestine is mainly by the superior and inferior mesenteric arteries. The internal iliac arteries supply the rectum and anus. Venous drainage is mainly by the superior and inferior mesenteric veins, and the rectum and anus are drained by the internal iliac veins. The nerves supplying the large intestine are via the sympathetic and parasympathetic nerves. The external anal sphincter is under voluntary control and is supplied by motor nerves from the spinal cord (Siegfried 2002; Ellis 2004).

Caecum

The small intestine terminates at the posteromedial aspect of the caecum. The caecum is fixed to the right side near the iliac crest. At the opening to the caecum there is a fold of mucous membrane known as the ileocaecal valve, which allows the passage of materials from the small intestine into the large intestine and prevents the reflux of contents from the colon back into the ileum. The contents of the colon are heavily colonised by bacteria whereas the small intestine is relatively free of microbes. The caecum is a dilated portion and has been described as a blind pouch approximately 6 cm in width and 8 cm in length. It is continuous with the ascending colon superiorly and has a blind end inferiorly. Attached to the caecum is a coiled tube closed at one end called the vermiform appendix. It is usually 8–13 cm in length although this can vary from 2.5 cm to 23 cm and has the same structure as the walls of the colon; however, it contains more lymphatic tissue (Moore & Dalley 1999).

Colon

Ascending colon
The ascending colon is approximately 15 cm long and joins the caecum at the ileocaecal junction. The ascending colon is covered with peritoneum anteriorly and on both sides, however, its posterior surface is devoid of peritoneum. It ascends on the right side of the abdomen to the level of the liver where it bends acutely to the left. At this point it forms the right colic or hepatic flexure and then continues as the transverse colon (Thibodeau & Patton 2002).

Transverse colon
This is a loop of colon approximately 45 cm long that continues from the left hepatic flexure across to the left side of the abdomen to the left colic flexure. It passes in front of the stomach and duodenum and then curves beneath the lower part of the spleen on the left side as the left colic or splenic flexure and then passes acutely downward as the descending colon (Watson 2000).

Descending colon
This section of the colon passes downwards on the left side of the abdomen to the level of the iliac crest. It is approximately

25 cm in length. The descending colon is narrower and more dorsally situated than the ascending colon.

Sigmoid colon

The sigmoid colon begins near the iliac crest and is approximately 36 cm long. It ends at the centre of the mid-sacrum, where it becomes the rectum at about the level of the third sacral vertebra. It is mobile and is completely covered by peritoneum and attached to the pelvic walls in an inverted V shape.

Rectum

The rectum is approximately 13 cm in length and begins where the colon loses its mesentery. It lies in the posterior aspect of the pelvis and ends 2–3 cm anteroinferiorly to the tip of the coccyx, where it bends downwards to form the anal canal (Tortora & Grabowski 2002).

Anal canal

This is the terminal segment of the large intestine and is approximately 4 cm in length opening to the exterior as the anus. The mucous membrane of the anal canal is arranged in longitudinal folds that contain a network of arteries and veins. The anus remains closed at rest. The anal canal corresponds anteriorly to the bulb of the penis in males and to the lower vagina in females and posteriorly it is related to the coccyx. The internal anal sphincter is composed of smooth muscle and is the lower of the two sphincters. It is about 2.5 cm long and can be palpated during rectal examination. It controls the upper two-thirds of the anal canal. The external sphincter is made up of skeletal muscle and is normally closed except during elimination of faeces. The nerve supply is from the perineal branch of the fourth sacral nerve and the inferior rectal nerves (Martini 2004).

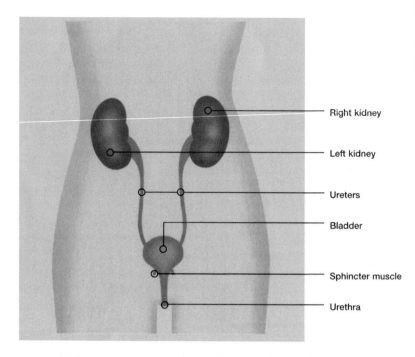

Right kidney

Left kidney

Ureters

Bladder

Sphincter muscle

Urethra

Fig. 1.2 The urinary system. Reproduced with kind permission of Coloplast Ltd from *An Introduction to Stoma Care* 2000

URINARY SYSTEM

The urinary system consists of the kidneys, ureters, bladder and urethra (Fig. 1.2). It has three major functions:

- excretion;
- elimination;
- homoeostatic regulation of the solute concentration of the blood plasma.

Kidneys

The kidneys are situated on either side of the vertebral column and they lie retroperitoneally between the 12th thoracic and

3rd lumbar vertebrae. The left kidney lies slightly superior to the right kidney and it is also slightly longer.

The kidneys are bean-shaped, and approximately 10–12 cm in length, 5–7 cm wide and 2–5 cm thick. The blood supply, nerves and lymphatic vessels enter and exit at the hilum.

The superior surface of the kidney is capped by the adrenal gland. Each kidney is surrounded by three layers.

(1) *Renal capsule:* this is a layer of collagen fibres that covers the outer surface of the entire organ.
(2) *Fat:* this keeps the kidney in place and surrounds the renal capsule.
(3) *Renal fascia:* this is a dense fibrous outer layer that also secures the kidney to the posterior abdominal wall and to the surrounding structures (Ross *et al.* 2001).

The kidney itself is made up of two layers, the cortex and the medulla. The cortex is the outer layer and the medulla is the inner layer. Within the medulla there are 8–18 distinct conical or triangular structures called the renal pyramids. The base of each pyramid is turned towards the cortex and the tip of the pyramid is directed towards the renal sinus. The tips of the pyramids are referred to as the renal papillae. The pyramids are separated from each other by bands of cortical tissue called the renal columns. The renal cortex and the pyramids together make up the parenchyma. The parenchyma consists of approximately 1.25 million nephrons, which are the functional units of the kidney as they form urine and help regulate the composition of the blood (Raferty 2000; Tucker 2002; Martini 2004)

Nephron

The nephron is the functional unit of the kidney. It is responsible for filtration of the blood and for the re-absorption of water and salts and the absorption of glucose. About 1.25 million nephrons can be found in the cortex. The nephron consists of a renal tubule and a renal corpuscle. The tubule is approximately 50 mm in length and consists of the convoluted tubule and the loop of Henle. The renal corpuscle is made up of the Bowman's capsule and the capillary network of the glomerulus (Tucker 2002).

Blood and nerve supply of the kidney

The right and left renal arteries transport about 20–25% of the total cardiac output and approximately 1200 ml will pass through the kidney each minute. As the renal artery enters the renal sinus, it divides into the five segmental arteries, which then subdivide into a series of interlobar arteries that radiate outwards and between the renal columns. At the base of the renal pyramids the arteries arch between the medulla and the cortex and are known as the arcuate arteries. These divide again to form the interlobular arteries. The interlobular arteries enter the renal cortex and become efferent arterioles which deliver blood to the capillaries known as peritubular capillaries.

Blood exits the kidney via the peritubular venules which then join the interlobular veins. These drain through the arcuate veins into the interlobar veins, which, in turn, join the segmental veins. The segmental veins join the renal vein which leaves the kidney at the hilum (Ellis 2004).

Nerve supply of the kidney

The nerve supply to the kidneys is from the renal nerves, which are derived from the renal plexus of the sympathetic division of the autonomic nervous system. The nerves enter the kidney at the hilum and run alongside the blood supply to reach the individual nephrons. The nerves regulate the circulation of blood in the kidneys by controlling the size of the arterioles (Martini 2004).

Ureters

The ureters are muscular tubes that link the kidneys to the bladder. They are approximately 30 cm in length and 3 mm in diameter. They consist of three layers: an inner layer of transitional epithelium, a middle layer made up of longitudinal and circular bands of smooth muscle and an outer layer of connective tissue which is continuous with the renal capsule. There are slight differences in the ureters in men and women as they have to accommodate the position of the reproductive organs.

The ureters transport urine from the kidneys to the bladder. Urine is forced along the ureter due to peristaltic action. The ureters enter the bladder on the posterior wall and pass into the bladder at an oblique angle. This prevents backflow when the bladder contracts (Ross *et al.* 2001).

Bladder

The bladder is a hollow, muscular organ that collects and stores urine. It is situated in the lower part of the abdomen and is lined with a membrane called the urothelium. The cells of this membrane are called transitional cells or urothelial cells. The bladder wall has three layers: mucosa, submucosa and muscularis. The muscularis is made up of layers of longitudinal smooth muscle with a circular layer sandwiched in between. This muscle layer is known as the detrusor muscle, and it is this mucle that contracts to expel urine from the bladder and into the urethra.

The bladder initally stores urine, however, afferent fibres in the pelvic nerves carry impulses to the spinal cord, which, in turn, sends messages to the thalamus and then along projection fibres to the cerebral cortex. At this point you become aware that your bladder requires emptying. The muscle of the bladder can then be contracted to force urine out of the body through a tube called the urethra (Ellis 2004).

Urethra

The urethra extends from the neck of the bladder to the exterior of the body. In women, the urethra is a very short tube, in front of the vagina, approximately 4 cm in length. In men, the tube is considerably longer, 18–20 cm long; it needs to be longer as it has to pass through the prostate gland and the length of the penis. It is made up of stratified epithelium (Ross *et al.* 2001; Thibodeau & Patton 2002; Martini 2004).

REFERENCES

Ellis, H. (2004) *Clinical Anatomy. A Revision and Applied Anatomy for Clinical Students.* Blackwell Science, Oxford.

Keshav, S. (2003) *The Gastrointestinal System at a Glance.* Blackwell Science, Oxford.

Kumar, P. & Clark, M. (1998) *Clinical Medicine*, 4th edn. W.B. Saunders, Edinburgh.

Lehne, T. (1998) The mouth and salivary glands. In: D.J. Weatherall, J.G. Ledingham & D.A. Warrell, eds. *Oxford Textbook of Medicine*, 3rd edn. Oxford University Press, Oxford.

Martini, F.H. (2004) *Fundamentals of Anatomy and Physiology.* Benjamin Cummings, San Fransisco.

Moore, K. & Dalley, A.F., eds. (1999) *Clinically Orientated Anatomy.* Lippincott Williams & Wilkins, Philadelphia.

Page, M., ed. (2001) *The Human Body.* Dorling Kindersley, London.

Raferty, A.T., ed. (2000) *Applied Science for Basic Surgical Training.* Churchill Livingstone, Edinburgh.

Ross, J.S., Wilson, R.J.W., Waugh, A. & Grant, A. (2001) *Ross and Wilson Anatomy and Physiology in Health and Illness*, 10th edn. Churchill Livingstone, Edinburgh.

Siegfried, D.R. (2002) *Anatomy and Physiology for Dummies.* John Wiley & Sons Inc, Columbia.

Thibodeau, G. & Patton, K.T. (2002) *Anatomy and Physiology*, 5th edn. C.V. Mosby, New York.

Tortora, G.J. & Grabowski, S.R. (2002) *Principles of Anatomy and Physiology*, 10th edn. John Wiley & Sons Inc, Columbia.

Tucker, L. (2002) *An Introductory Guide to Anatomy and Physiology*, revised edn. Holistic Therapy Books, Cambridge.

Watson, R. (2000) *Anatomy and Physiology for Nurses*, 11th edn. Baillère Tindall, Royal College of Nursing, Edinburgh.

Faecal and Urinary Stomas and the Restorative Surgical Procedures Developed to Avoid Stoma Formation

2

Anthony McGrath & Theresa Porrett

INTRODUCTION

A stoma is an artificial opening in the bowel, created by a surgeon to divert the flow of faeces and/or urine. The word stoma comes from the Greek for mouth or opening (Black 1997a). The aim of this chapter is to increase the reader's knowledge and understanding of the types of stoma formed in the UK today, and to raise awareness of the complex restorative procedures that patients undergo in an effort to avoid a permanent stoma. The different types of stoma will be described and the sites they can be found on the abdomen. This chapter also discusses the issues that surround both permanent and temporary stomas and describes a number of restorative 'pouch' procedures.

LEARNING OBJECTIVES

By the end of this chapter the reader should be able to:

❏ differentiate between the different types of stoma formed;
❏ apply this knowledge to plan and provide effective care for patients undergoing stoma formation;
❏ discuss the variety of restorative procedures available.

There are approximately 80 000–100 000 people at any one time in the UK with a stoma (Devlin *et al.* 1971; Coloplast 1995) (see Table 2.1). In approximately 65% of patients who have a stoma formed it will be permanent (Black 1997b,c). To form a stoma the bowel (ileum or colon) is surgically divided and the ends

Table 2.1 Stomal incidence (Black 1997a, c; Coloplast 1995)

Type of stoma	Existing numbers (approx)	Annual incidence (approx)
Colostomy	40 000	11 000
Ileostomy	15 000	2 000
Urostomy	7 500	1 000

brought to the surface of the abdominal wall as a loop or end stoma. When formed stomas should appear pinkish red (very similar to the inside of the mouth). There are three main types of stoma:

- colostomy;
- ileostomy;
- urostomy.

PERMANENT AND TEMPORARY STOMAS

A stoma may be temporary or permanent. A temporary stoma is most often created to divert faeces away from an operation site (anastomosis) to allow healing to occur without irritation or to provide an outlet for faeces when an obstruction is present. This stoma can then be reversed by the surgeon with minimal or no loss of intestinal function. A permanent stoma implies that the bowel cannot be reconnected. Therefore the patient will never have a 'normal' functioning bowel again. A permanent stoma may be required when a disease, or its treatment, leads to loss of normal intestinal function. The most common conditions where a permanent stoma is required are cancer of the rectum and inflammatory bowel disease.

PRINCIPLES OF STOMA FORMING SURGERY

- Adequate blood supply to the mobilised bowel forming the stoma must be maintained otherwise the stoma can become necrotic.

- The bowel forming the stoma must not be placed under tension when being brought to the surface of the abdominal wall (this can cause retraction).
- The laparotomy incision must be kept away from the position of the stoma (as scars can cause appliance adherence and leakage problems).
- Wherever possible the patient should have the optimum site for the stoma marked before the operation (otherwise patients may have problems in managing the stoma) (see Chapter 4).

COLOSTOMY

When the large bowel is unable to function normally because of disease or injury, or needs to rest from normal function, the body must have another way to eliminate faeces. A colostomy is an opening made into the large bowel during surgery and the bowel is then brought through the abdominal wall onto the skin. This provides a new path for faeces and flatus to exit the body. A colostomy is created to treat various disorders of the large intestine such as inflammatory bowel disease, cancer, obstruction, diverticular disease, ischaemia, or traumatic injury (see Fig. 3.1 in Chapter 3). A colostomy may be temporary or permanent.

Permanent colostomy

A permanent colostomy is also referred to as an end or terminal colostomy. It is most commonly situated in the left iliac fossa. An incision is made in the abdominal wall through the muscle layers and into the peritoneum. The bowel is passed through the abdominal wall to the skin and then sutured into place. An end colostomy is usually formed from the descending or sigmoid colon. The rectum and section of the bowel beyond the stoma are usually removed. The resultant stoma is approximately 2.5 cm wide and protrudes about 0.5–1 cm above the abdominal surface (Black 2000).

Patients with a permanent colostomy will find that their stool remains formed as most of the water has been absorbed by the colon as normal. They may find that they now pass stool once or twice daily. The most common surgical procedures associated with a permanent colostomy are an abdominoperineal excision of the rectum and Hartmann's procedure (see Chapter 3).

Temporary colostomy

Temporary colostomies are created to divert stool from injured or diseased portions of the large intestine, allowing rest and healing. A temporary colostomy can be either a loop colostomy or a double-barrel colostomy.

Loop colostomy

A loop colostomy may be constructed in the sigmoid or transverse colon. It is created by bringing a loop of bowel through an incision in the abdominal wall. An incision is made in the bowel to allow the passage of faeces through the loop colostomy. A rod is usually placed under the loop of bowel but on top of the skin. The rod supports the loop of bowel and prevents retraction into the abdomen. The rod is usually removed approximately three to five days after surgery. The output from a loop colostomy will depend on which part of the colon was used. If the loop was made in the transverse colon the stool will be loose and semi-formed. A loop formed from sigmoid colon will result in a more formed stool as more water will have been absorbed (Black 2000).

Double-barrel colostomy

This type of colostomy involves the creation of two separate stomas on the abdominal wall. Two sections of the descending or sigmoid colon are used. The incision is usually made in the left iliac fossa. The output is usually formed.

ILEOSTOMY

An ileostomy involves bringing the ileum to the abdominal surface. It is usually sited in the right iliac fossa. There are two types of ileostomy: an end ileostomy and a loop ileostomy.

End ileostomy

An end ileostomy involves the removal of the large bowel. The ileum is brought to the surface of the abdominal wall and everted to form a spout. The spout is usually 3–5 cm in length. This spouted ileostomy is often referred to as a Brooke ileostomy after the surgeon, Brian Brooke, who invented the procedure. Patients do not have any control over their bowel movements and the motions are very soft and porridge- or fluid-like. As there is no control over bowel movements a drainable bag is used to collect body waste products. The bag is emptied as often as necessary, usually between six and eight times a day (Black 2000).

Loop ileostomy

A loop ileostomy is created when a loop of ileum is brought out onto the abdomen in the right iliac fossa. It is a temporary stoma and is usually used to assist the large bowel to heal. It is often used after surgery such as an anterior resection (see Chapter 3).

A loop ileostomy is more commonly used than a loop colostomy to defunction the colon because it is less bulky and can be sited lower than a loop colostomy and therefore is easier to manage. A loop ileostomy is formed in a similar way to a loop colostomy. A section of ileum is brought to the surface of the abdominal wall; this loop of bowel is supported by a plastic rod, which is removed three to five days following surgery. The loop of ileum is cut, leaving only about a third of its circumference joined together. The functioning or proximal end is spouted and the distal limb is sutured flat to the skin.

RESTORATIVE PROCEDURES

Restorative procedures are complex, staged surgical procedures which have the aim of avoiding a permanent stoma.
However supported and able patients are to resume their
normal life with a stoma, some will feel stigmatised by
society's perception of stomas and our focus on the ideal or
perfect body. In 1978, Dudley wrote, 'However managed,
however we delude ourselves, a permanent potentially incontinent stoma is an affront difficult to bear, so that I marvel that
we and our patients have put up with it for so long.' Given
the patient demand for continent procedures, it is apparent
that this feeling holds true for many today. Consequently, the
number of new stomas formed has not changed considerably
over the past three decades, but what has changed is the proportion of permanent versus temporary stomas: approximately 45% of stomas are temporary in nature (Black 1997c).
Such complex surgical procedures are associated with significant complications and physical and psychological morbidity
(Porrett 1996). The demand for all types of continent and
restorative procedures is increasing as an ever greater number
of patients seek an alternative to a permanent stoma (Salter
1996) and an escape from social stigma.

Ileo-anal pouch (restorative proctocolectomy)

Developed in 1978 (Parks & Nicholls 1978), restorative proctocolectomy is suitable for those with familial adenomatous
polyposis and ulcerative colitis. It involves resection of the
colon and proximal rectum and construction of an ileal pouch
with an ileo-anal anastomosis. The ileo-anal pouch is often
referred to as a Parks' pouch and can also be described by it
shape: J-pouch, S-pouch and W-pouch. The J-shaped pouch is
the most commonly performed as it can be formed using
modern stapling guns (Porrett 1996) (Fig. 2.1). Following
removal of the anal canal and rectum a reservoir (pouch) is
constructed from the small intestine (ileum) and connected to
the sphincter muscles (the muscle that surround the anus).

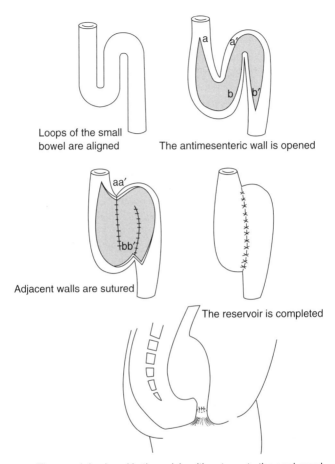

Loops of the small bowel are aligned

The antimesenteric wall is opened

Adjacent walls are sutured

The reservoir is completed

The pouch is placed in the pelvis with sutures to the anal canal

Fig. 2.1 Construction of a Parks' pouch. Reproduced with kind permission of Coloplast Ltd from *An Introduction to Stoma Care* 2000

Although this procedure can be performed in one stage it is not uncommon for a temporary loop ileostomy to be formed to protect the pouch anastomosis. This can then be closed at around three months as long as there is no anastomotic leak (patients have a gastrograffin enema to ensure no leakage from the pouch). Once the loop ileostomy is closed the pouch functions as a neo-rectum and stores faecal fluid. As the colon has been removed the patient will pass porridge-like stools and the pouch can be active between two and eight times during the day and in some patients once or twice at night (Porrett 1996). So although a permanent stoma is avoided this is not a return to normal bowel function, and therefore patients require very careful pre-operative counselling to ensure they realise the potential disadvantages of this procedure (Mortensen 1993; Black 2000).

Pouchitis is the commonest complication of this surgery and is an inflammation of the pouch. This inflammation causes symptoms which are similar to those of ulcerative colitis, loose bloody stools, frequency of defaecation and pain. Pouchitis can be treated using a number of medical regimens similar to those used to treat ulcerative colitis.

Kock pouch

For patients who have already undergone a panproctocolectomy (removal of the large colon and rectum) Kock continent ileostomy is an option. This procedure is also suitable for patients who are suffering from ulcerative colitis and familial adenomatous polyposis. It was first devised by Professor Nils Kock in 1969 in which he described the formation of an internal reservoir (Black 2000). The pouch is formed from the terminal ileum, approximately 45 cm is used to construct it. Two loops of ileum are sewn together to form the reservoir. The surgeon will aim to produce a pouch with a capacity of 500–1000 ml. A nipple valve is constructed by intussuscepting approximately 15 cm of the ileum into the pouch. This is then secured in place and has an opening on the right iliac fossa. The patient can empty the reservoir by passing a catheter into the pouch four to five times daily and allowing the faeces to drain. This procedure gives patients more control over elimination. The main advantage of this procedure is that it has an internal pouch, so the need for an appliance is removed, and the stoma can be sited lower down on the abdomen and is therefore less noticeable than a conventionally sited stoma. However, there is a risk that the valve will become displaced or will cease to function correctly. This type of pouch has become less popular since the advent of ileo-anal pouch surgery.

Gracilis neo-sphincter

Gracilis neo-sphincter is a procedure for patients who have undergone abdominal surgery that resulted in permanent stoma formation but who find life with a permanent stoma unmanageable. The surgery is primarily suitable for patients with faecal incontinence where previous surgery has failed to restore continence, those in whom the sphincter has been removed following surgery such as abdomino-perineal resection of rectum or panproctocolectomy or those in whom the sphincter muscle is absent, conditions such as imperforate anus (Black 2000).

The procedure is usually undertaken in two stages. Stage 1 involves transferring the gracilis muscle from the inner thigh and tunnelling it under the skin and wrapping it around the anal canal (Stuchfield & Eccersley 1999). At this time a loop ileostomy is fashioned to minimise the risk of faecal contamination. The gracilis muscle is designed for short contractions rather than sustained contraction, and therefore a technique has been developed which converts the muscle to a fatigue-resistant muscle allowing it to function as the internal anal sphincter does, remaining contracted for long periods of time. This process involves electrically stimulating the muscle over a period of weeks, with the period of stimulation being increased gradually. During stage 1 of the procedure an electrode plate is attached over the nerve supply to the gracilis muscle and a stimulator is implanted subcutaneously in the abdominal wall. The temporary stoma is closed in stage 2 of the procedure when all wounds have healed and the conver-

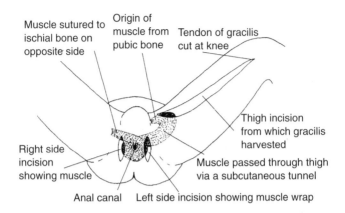

Muscle sutured to ischial bone on opposite side

Origin of muscle from pubic bone

Tendon of gracilis cut at knee

Thigh incision from which gracilis harvested

Right side incision showing muscle

Muscle passed through thigh via a subcutaneous tunnel

Anal canal   Left side incision showing muscle wrap

Fig. 2.2 Formation of gracilis neo-sphincter showing incisions and muscle wrap. Reproduced with kind permission of Whurr Publishers from Porrett & Daniel 1999

sion of the muscle has been completed. Patients are then taught to use the stimulator. When stimulated the muscle occludes the anal canal and when the stimulator is turned off the muscle relaxes allowing defaecation (Fig. 2.2).

Some patients have problems with defaecation and need to use laxatives or suppositories; others experience faecal soiling and may need to use pads. Throughout the procedure (Stuchfield & Eccersley 1999) and follow-up the patient requires a great deal of support and education. Consequently, the surgery is performed in specialist centres only.

Urostomy

Urostomy is the general term for the diversion of the urinary tract. It is usually performed in patients who have a diseased or defective bladder. The surgeon creates a passageway for urine to pass from the kidneys to the outside of the body through a stoma. The main reasons for urinary diversion are:

- cancer of the bladder;
- neuropathic bladder;
- urinary incontinence (Black 2000).

Ileal conduit

The surgeon will usually remove the bladder, however, this is dependent on the underlying condition. First described by Bricker (1950), the ileal conduit is the most common type of urinary diversion (Harvey 1997). A section of ileum is resected with its blood supply (close to the ileocaecal valve), approximately 10–20 cm. One end of this resected ileum is sutured closed and the two ureters are then anastomosed into this loop of ileum. The other end is then brought out onto the skin as an everted spouted stoma (it looks exactly like an ileostomy). Urine drains almost constantly from the kidneys, down the ureters into the isolated ileum and out of the spouted stoma into an appliance.

Continent urinary diversions

There are a number of procedures that aim to replace or rebuild the body's urinary system. They generally consist of three parts: a reservoir for urine, a channel to let the urine out, and a continence mechanism to retain urine (Leaver 1996). In the UK, the most commonly performed urinary diversion is called the Mitrofanoff pouch and is suitable for patients with congenital abnormalities, neuropathic bladder, bladder trauma, carcinoma of the bladder and urinary incontinence (see Table 3.1 in Chapter 3, Woodhouse 1991). The procedure involves major surgery and the patient needs to be well motivated and committed to the resultant ongoing self-catheterisation of the pouch.

Surgery can take up to five hours and has a high complication rate with some patients requiring a 48-hour postoperative stay in a high dependency unit (Leaver 1996). Basically the surgery involves taking a section of bowel to form a pouch (sometimes the pouch can be made of bladder or bladder augmented by bowel). The ureters are anastomosed to the pouch. The pouch is then connected to the abdominal wall by a channel (such as the appendix, or fallopian tube). This channel is prevented from leaking urine by the creation of a non-return 'flap' valve (Leaver 1997). A catheter is inserted into the pouch to drain it. Once formed the 'new' bladder must be kept empty of urine for about six weeks after surgery and this involves a stoma catheter, a suprapubic catheter and ureteric stents to the kidney. Prior to discharge from hospital the ureteric stents and suprapubic catheter are removed leaving only the stomal catheter (Leaver 1997). Patients are discharged with this catheter on free drainage for approximately six weeks. At this stage patients are re-admitted to hospital and the pouch is expanded to assess its capacity. Patients are taught to intermittently catheterise the pouch to drain urine.

There are some perceived advantages of restorative procedures versus stoma forming surgery:

- no change in body image as no appliance and no protruding stoma;
- no perceived social or sporting restrictions;
- a perception that this is a return to 'normal' bodily function;
- no stigma.

Although these are obvious advantages for patients, restorative surgery procedures are not suitable for everybody. Patients have to be particularly motivated and compliant with the need for long-term follow-up. They must also accept the higher complication rate in comparison with more standard stoma forming operations.

SELF-EVALUATION QUESTIONS AND ANSWERS

Questions

1. A complication of ileo-anal pouch surgery might be:
   A. Constipation
   B. Pouchitis

   C. Nausea

   D. Limited physical activity

2. The gracilis neo-sphincter procedure is not performed for which of the following conditions:

   A. Faecal incontinence

   B. Urinary incontinence

   C. Imperforate anus

   D. Previous rectal cancer in which surgery has removed the anal sphincters

3. Which of the following statements is true? Following a Mitrofanoff pouch procedure:

   A. Ureteric stents are removed after approximately two weeks but the stomal catheter is left in place for six weeks

   B. The bladder is irrigated daily

   C. Urine is passed in the normal way

   D. The bladder is removed and a permanent stoma is formed

4. The ileo-anal pouch is a surgical option for patients with:

   A. Crohn's disease

   B. Diverticulitis

   C. Recurrent bowel cancer

   D. Ulcerative colitis and familial adenomatous polyposis (FAP)

5. A loop ileostomy is performed to protect the bowel and allow an anastomosis to heal.
    True or false?

6. The end colostomy formed following a Hartmann's procedure can never be closed.
    True or false?

7. Transverse loop colostomies produce formed stool and function once a day.
    True or false?

8. An ileostomy is flush with the skin.
    True or false?

9. An end ileostomy following a proctocolectomy is a permanent stoma.
    True or false?

Answers

1. B	6. False
2. B	7. False
3. A	8. False
4. D	9. True
5. True	

REFERENCES

Black, P. (1997a) *Practical stoma care. Nursing Standard* **11**, 49–55.

Black, P. (1997b) Practical stoma care: a community approach. *British Journal of Community Health Nursing* **2**, 249–53.

Black, P. (1997c) Life carries on: stoma aftercare. *Practice Nursing* **8**, 29–32.

Black, P. (2000) *Holistic Stoma Care*. Ballière Tindall, London.

Bricker, E.M. (1950) Bladder substitution after pelvic evisceration. *Surgical Clinics of North America* **30**, 1151.

Coloplast Ltd (1995) *Ostomy and Ostomy Patients*. Coloplast Ltd, Peterborough.

Devlin, H.B., Plant, J.A. & Griffin, M. (1971) Aftermath of surgery for anorectal cancer. *British Medical Journal* **3**, 413–18.

Dudley, H.A.F. (1978) If I had carcinoma of the middle third of the rectum. *British Medical Journal* **1**, 1035–67.

Harvey, H. (1997) Urological stomas. In: S. Fillingham & J. Douglas, eds. *Urological Nursing*. Ballière Tindall, London.

Leaver, R.B. (1996) Continent urinary diversions – the Mitrofanoff principle. In: C. Myers, ed. *Stoma Care Nursing – A Patient Centred Approach*. Arnold, London.

Leaver, R.B. (1997) Reconstructive surgery for the promotion of continence. In: S. Fillingham & J. Douglas, eds. *Urological Nursing*. Ballière Tindall, London.

Mortensen, N. (1993) Patient selection for restorative proctocolectomy. In: R.J. Nichols, D. Bartolo and N. Mortensen, eds. *Restorative Proctocolectomy*. Blackwell Science, Oxford.

Parks, A.G. & Nicholls, R.J. (1978) Proctocolectomy without ileostomy for ulcerative colitis. *British Medical Journal* **ii**, 85–8.

Porrett, T. (1996) *Restorative proctocolectomy*. In: C. Mayers, ed. *Stoma Care Nursing – A Patient Centred Approach*. Arnold, London.

Salter, M. (1996) Advances in ileostomy care. *Nursing Standard* **11**, 49–55.

Stuchfield, B. & Eccersley, A. (1999) The modern management of faecal incontinence. In: T. Porrett & N. Daniel, eds. *Essential Coloproctology for Nurses.* Whurr Publishers, London.

Woodhouse, C.R.J. (1991) The Mitrofanoff principle for continent urinary diversion. *World Council of Enterostomal Therapists Journal* **11**, 12–15.

3 Rationale for Stoma Formation and Common Surgical Procedures

Anthony McGrath & Theresa Porrett

INTRODUCTION

This chapter will explore some of the reasons why patients undergo stoma forming surgery and will provide an insight into the various conditions and diseases and how they affect the patient. The most common surgical procedures are also discussed.

LEARNING OUTCOMES

By reading this chapter the reader will have:

❏ an understanding of the various pathological conditions that may require surgery and result in stoma formation;
❏ an understanding of Crohn's disease and ulcerative colitis;
❏ an appreciation of the surgical procedures which form temporary and permanent stomas.

Patients may undergo stoma forming surgery for a number of reasons (see Table 3.1). These include:

- inflammatory bowel disease;
- diverticular disease;
- familial adenomatous polyposis;
- carcinoma of the bladder;
- carcinoma of the bowel;
- traumatic injury to the abdominal area;
- inadequate blood flow to the bowel;
- incontinence;
- obstruction.

Table 3.1 Conditions which may result in stoma formation

Conditions which may result in stoma formation	Ileostomy		Colostomy		Urostomy
	Permanent	Temporary	Permanent	Temporary	
Sigmoid colon cancer		✓	✓	✓	
Colon cancer		✓			
Rectal cancer		✓	✓	✓	
Crohn's disease	✓	✓	✓	✓	
Diverticular disease			✓	✓	
Irradiation damage	✓				✓
Bowel ischaemia	✓				
Faecal incontinence			✓		
Volvulus				✓	
Trauma		✓		✓	✓
Congenital abnormalities			✓	✓	✓
Hirschsprung's disease		✓	✓	✓	
Ulcerative colitis	✓				
Constipation			✓		
Familial adenomatous polyposis	✓				
Bladder cancer					✓
Urethral cancer					✓
Urinary fistulae					✓
Spinal lesions					✓
Urinary incontinence					✓

INFLAMMATORY BOWEL DISEASE

Inflammatory bowel disease (IBD) refers to two chronic conditions, ulcerative colitis and Crohn's disease. The peak age of onset of both diseases occurs in the 20–40 year age group with a second peak in the 65 years and above age group (Black 2000). Women appear to be affected more than men. There appears to be a genetic link to these disorders and in the UK both disorders occur at a higher rate in the Jewish community than in the indigenous population. Initially, Crohn's disease affected mainly the white population, however, is becoming more common in Asian immigrants to the UK.

The prevalence for both disorders (i.e. the number of people affected in a population at any given time) is as follows:

- ulcerative colitis – 160 per 100 000;
- Crohn's disease – 50 per 100 000 (Kamm 1996).

Ulcerative colitis

Ulcerative colitis is a chronic inflammatory disorder that affects the large bowel although in some cases the distal part of the terminal ileum can be affected (backwash ileitis). It affects the mucosa of the colon and rectum causing swelling, inflammation and ulceration. Patients have bouts of bloody diarrhoea. Ulcerative colitis is characterised by widespread ulceration of the superficial layers of the large bowel. In the majority of cases, it begins in the rectum and then extends proximally in a continuous fashion. It is a disease characterised by relapses and remissions. Systemic problems associated with ulcerative colitis are: arthritis, erythema nodosum (painful swellings, particularly on the lower legs), ankylosing spondylitis (stiffness and loss of spinal movement) and pyoderma gangrenosum (painful ulcers) (Turnburg 1989). Long term, patients may experience liver damage and sclerosing cholangitis (fibrosing inflammation of bile ducts), and they are known to be at an increased risk of developing cancer of the colon.

Crohn's disease

Crohn's disease was first described in 1932 by Dr Crohn as occurring in the terminal ileum. However, we now know that Crohn's disease occurs most commonly in the ileocaecal region but can occur anywhere from the mouth to the anus. Crohn's disease is a chronic, progressive, granulomatous inflammatory disorder. It is transmural, i.e. affects the full thickness of the intestinal wall and causes inflammation and thickening of the bowel. Often this inflammation causes a narrowing of the lumen (stricture). Crohn's disease is characterised by 'skip lesions', i.e. areas of diseased bowel with healthy areas in between (Joels 1999). The inflammation may involve the entire thickness of the bowel wall, leading to severe ulceration and the formation of fistulae. The symptoms of Crohn's can be non-specific and vary according to the area of bowel affected, but most commonly include:

- diarrhoea and bleeding, although bleeding is less common than in ulcerative colitis;
- cramping abdominal pain;
- subacute gastrointestinal obstruction;
- anorexia and weight loss;
- fever;
- anal and perianal lesions (skin tags, abscesses and fistulae) (Black 2000).

AETIOLOGY OF IBD

The causes of ulcerative colitis and Crohn's disease remain unknown, however, a variety of theories have been put forward.

- Bacterial and viral infections: These are generally thought to be one of the multifactorial elements that are involved in the aetiology of IBD. There has been much research into the finding of a direct relation between a microbial pathogen and IBD. However, recent reports suggest that it is not a specific infection that causes IBD, but rather enteric pathogens cause the initial onset of IBD and episodes of relapse (Stallmach & Carstens 2002). It has been suggested that these infections initiate a cascade of inflammatory events leading to a chronic inflammatory response in genetically susceptible hosts (Sartor 1993). The measles virus has also been linked with the development of Crohn's disease (Thompson 1995). However, recent studies found neither epidemiologic nor molecular evidence supporting an aetiological or pathogenic link between the measles virus and Crohn's disease (Afzal *et al.* 1998; Peltola *et al.* 1998). The majority of research has focused on the harmful effects of bacteria, however, there is now increasing interest in the benefits of manipulating normal intestinal flora with probiotics. It is believed that elements of the flora down-regulate inflammation (Katz *et al.* 1999).

- Genetic predisposition: In patients with ulcerative colitis the chances of a sibling, parent or child having the condition as well is between 1 in 15 and 1 in 10. This is about 50 times the risk of the general population. In identical twins, if one has Crohn's the other has a 50% chance of developing the disease (Forbes 2002).

- Smoking: On one hand this is seen to be beneficial especially in ulcerative colitis and is thought to prevent disease recurrence. However, in patients with Crohn's it causes problems and is associated with disease 'flare-ups' (Pullan 1996).

- Diet: It is thought that diet has a role in causing IBD and some researchers have looked at the western diet high in processed foods as being a cause. This theory is backed up by the fact that some patients have had success with dietary changes such as the exclusion of dairy products in ulcerative colitis. In Crohn's disease the use of elemental feeds (a liquid feed with all the nutrients needed in a 'predigested' form thus absorbed through the small intestine) has been shown to be beneficial. It brings about symptomatic relief while simultaneously addressing the often compromised nutritional state of many patients (Wight & Scott 1997).

- Immunological factors: Many of the symptoms that patients present with are similar to those in conditions that are known to be autoimmune disorders such rheumatoid arthritis. It has been found in IBD that T cell lymphocyte regulation is disturbed and there is also an increased production of cytokines, leukotrienes and prostaglandins, which are responsible for tissue damage.

MEDICAL MANAGEMENT OF IBD

As the aetiology of IBD is unknown, medical treatment is centred on symptom control and is dependent on the severity of the episode. The aim is to bring about a remission in the disease and to maintain this as long as possible. Corticosteroids (prednisolone) form the backbone of treatment in acute episodes as they help control the inflammation in the bowel. They can be given intravenously, orally or rectally. When a patient achieves remission they can be maintained on medications such as the 5-ASA drugs (sulfasalazine, mesalazine), which belong to the aminosalicylates (ASA) group (Forbes 2002).

Patients with mild to moderate exacerbations of ulcerative colitis can be treated as outpatients. Local disease of the rectum and sigmoid colon can often be managed by topical therapy with 5 ASA and steroids in the form of suppositories or foam enemas. However, hospital admission is usually required for severe attacks as they will probably require the administration of intravenous fluids and corticosteroids. Patients will require nutritional support as they tend to lose weight quickly and excessive protein losses can occur due to bleeding. When the patient is admitted they will require close observation because of the risk of toxic megacolon (extreme dilatation of the large intestine) and perforation causing peritonitis, which is an indication for an emergency operation (colectomy). Patients with Crohn's can be anaemic due to blood loss and they may require blood transfusion. If the patient does not respond to medical treatment the doctors will consider surgical intervention.

SURGICAL MANAGEMENT OF IBD

Surgical intervention is usually reserved for when medical management has failed. It is estimated that 20–30% of patients with ulcerative colitis will need surgical treatment, usually within the first five years of diagnosis. Surgery is reserved for the complications of Crohn's disease such as strictures, fistula formation, obstruction and severe haemorrhage. According to Becker (1999), patients with terminal ileum and colonic disease are more likely to require surgical intervention than those with disease confined to the colon or rectum.

Ulcerative colitis

There are several surgical options to treat ulcerative colitis and these include:

- total/subtotal colectomy and formation of ileostomy with preservation of the rectal stump;
- total colectomy and ileorectal anastomosis;
- panproctocolectomy and formation of permanent ileostomy;
- Restorative proctocolectomy (see Chapter 2).

Subtotal colectomy

The colon is removed, an end ileostomy is formed but the rectum is preserved allowing restorative surgery to be considered in the future. The rectal stump is often brought to the surface of the abdomen, at the lower end of the laparotomy wound (mucous fistula). Once the patient is well, ileo-anal pouch surgery can be discussed as an alternative to a permanent ileostomy, since having lived with an ileostomy patients can make a more informed decision about further surgery (Joels 1999, Table 3.1; Figure 3.1).

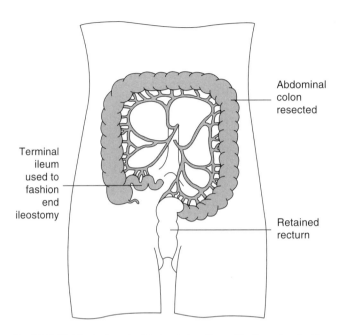

Fig. 3.1 Subtotal colectomy for fulminant ulcerative colitis. Reproduced with kind permission of Aventis Pharma UK Ltd from Thomas, *A Guide to Colorectal Surgery*, 2001

Total colectomy

In this procedure the whole colon is removed. The rectal stump is preserved and an end ileostomy formed. This is commonly performed as an emergency procedure in patients with fulminating colitis (extensive colitis which is not resolving on medical treatment and therefore there is a high risk of colonic perforation) or toxic megacolon. Once the patient has recovered from their surgery further restorative surgery can be discussed (ileo-anal pouch) (Black 2000, Table 3.1). Ileo-anal pouch surgery is discussed in Chapter 2.

Panproctocolectomy

Panproctocolectomy was the operation of choice for patients with ulcerative colitis from the 1950s until the introduction of the ileo-anal pouch procedure in the 1980s. It remains the main surgical procedure offered to patients with severe colonic/rectal and anal inflammatory bowel disease (Joels 1999). The surgery involves removing the colon, rectum and anal canal and forming a permanent ileostomy. The surgery has the advantage of curing the disease as all of the colon/rectum is removed but the disadvantages include delayed healing of the perineal wound (up to 25% of patients have an unhealed wound up to six months following the surgery) (Nicholls 1996, Table 3.1).

Crohn's disease

As Crohn's disease can affect the whole of the gastrointestinal tract, a cure by resecting the bowel is not possible. Therefore surgical intervention is directed at treating the complications of the disease such as strictures, fistulae or bowel obstruction. Depending on the extent of the diseased area and its site surgical intervention may or may not involve stoma formation. However, if the rectum and anus are badly affected a permanent colostomy or ileostomy may be required.

DIVERTICULAR DISEASE

Diverticula are small pouches (pockets) protruding from the bowel wall. They can occur in any part of the bowel; however they occur predominantly in the sigmoid colon. Asymptomatic diverticular disease is called diverticulosis. Many people are unaware that they have this condition. However, if the diverticula become inflamed it is called diverticulitis. Women appear to be affected more than men (Knowles & Lunniss 2003).

It has been estimated that by the age of 60 one-third of the population of the western world have diverticulosis (Schoetz 1993). It is believed that this high incidence is due to diet, a lack of dietary fibre being considered to be the main reason that the condition develops. Research has identified that many patients with this condition have a low intake of fruit, vegetables and bran, however, in contrast their meat intake is high (Sher *et al.* 1999). It is believed that the lack of fibre leads to high intraluminal pressures. This, in turn, causes the gut mucosa to herniate through the muscle wall. Faeces can then collect in the pouches leading to inflammation, abscess formation, perforation and fistula formation between the colon and the bladder, vagina or small bowel. Patients may also complain of pain, haemorrhage and stricture formation, however, diverticulitis rarely presents with bleeding only (Sher *et al.* 1999).

Signs and symptoms
Patients with diverticulitis present with bleeding, an altered bowel habit, pyrexia, flatulence, nausea and colicky type pain which is usually in the left iliac fossa and is relieved by defecation. In severe cases the inflamed diverticulum can perforate leading to peritonitis and the patient will require urgent surgical intervention and probable stoma formation.

Indications for surgery
Obstruction, abscess formation, fistula formation, perforation and repeated attacks are indications for surgery. If emergency surgery is required a Hartmann's procedure is most commonly performed.

Hartmann's procedure
In Hartmann's procedure the sigmoid colon and upper part of the rectum are excised. The rectal stump is over sewn and left in place, and the sigmoid colon is brought to the surface of the abdominal wall (on the left) as an end colostomy (Elcoat 1986). This procedure is usually performed for obstructing sigmoid cancers or perforated diverticular disease and therefore often takes place as an emergency operation with the patient acutely

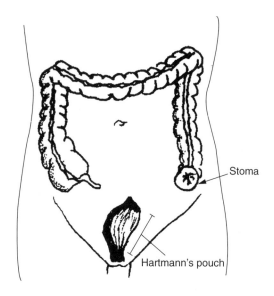

Fig. 3.2 The descending colostomy and closed rectal (Hartmann's) stump. Reproduced with kind permission of Whurr Publishers from Porrett & Daniel 1999

unwell with peritonitis. The procedure takes approximately one and a half hours and results in an end colostomy. Once the patient has recovered from surgery it is possible to restore bowel continence by joining the sigmoid colon to the rectal stump. Many patients are elderly and frail and therefore they decide not to undergo further major surgery (up to 60–70%) and continue with their colostomy (Knowles & Lunniss 2003) (Fig. 3.2; Table 3.1).

FAMILIAL ADENOMATOUS POLYPOSIS (FAP)

FAP is a rare hereditary disease that usually occurs in the teens and early twenties. It is an autosomal dominant condition caused by a mutation of the *APC* gene (Neale & Philips 2002).

Large numbers of adenomatous polyps grow in the colon. These polyps are pre-malignant and if left untreated they will develop into colonic cancer. The treatment of FAP is surgical and involves removing the colon. A proctocolectomy with permanent ileostomy, a colectomy with ileorectal anastomosis or a restorative proctocolectomy are most commonly performed. In most hospitals the ileo-anal pouch is the preferred approach for these young people as it allows removal of the entire colon and rectum but avoids a permanent stoma (Nogueras & McGannon 1999) (see Chapter 2).

As this is an inherited family disease it is important that the patient's family is also followed-up and screened for the condition. Patients will require lifelong regular follow-up and this is usually undertaken at a polyposis registry (there are a number in the UK). The oldest polyposis registry in the UK is at St Mark's Hospital and was founded in 1924 (Neale & Philips 2002). In each 'registry' an integrated team of doctors, nurses, genetic counsellors and social workers will plan care and follow-up and monitor entire families. One of the most important functions of the registry team is to facilitate compliance with surveillance (Nogueras & McGannon 1999).

COLORECTAL CANCER

This is the second commonest cause of cancer deaths in the UK. It affects all age groups, however, it is commoner in those individuals aged 55–70+ years. Patients aged 70+ make up 56% of all presentations (Hope *et al.* 1998). It can affect any part of the large bowel although it is more commonly found in the sigmoid colon and the rectum. Diet, IBD and a family history are linked with its development, however, the exact cause is still unclear. Some studies have demonstrated that a diet low in vegetables increases the risk of developing cancer.

In the majority of cases, colon cancer arises from an adenomatous polyp, over time this benign polyp becomes malignant (Weiss & Johnson 1999). As the malignancy grows it can spread circumferentially or into the lumen of the bowel eventually causing obstruction. The cancer will then spread further by infiltrating the wall of the bowel and into organs such as the liver via the lymphatic system and the blood.

Signs and symptoms

Colorectal cancers may develop and not cause any symptoms until they are at an advanced stage. Many patients will present in A&E with bowel obstruction, perforation and peritonitis. The symptoms of colorectal cancer include an altered bowel habit and bleeding. Patients may note that blood is mixed in with their stool and they may experience 'tenesmus'. Patients describe this as a constant painful feeling of wanting to open their bowels. When the doctors digitally examine the rectum they may note the presence of a mass. Blood tests may reveal a low haemoglobin level indicating blood loss.

Investigations and treatment

The patient may undergo the following tests:

- a colonoscopy;
- a barium enema;
- CT (computed tomography) scan;
- liver ultrasound;
- a chest x-ray;
- positron emission tomography (PET scanning). A PET scan is a metabolic imaging examination and can detect and stage most cancers and metastasis;
- magnetic resonance imaging (MRI) scanning (is used to stage rectal cancers);
- blood will be taken to check haemoglobin levels and liver function.

Following diagnosis the medical staff will discuss with the patient and their family the treatment options available to them; these will vary depending on the site and size of the tumour and also if there is any local or distant spread.

Treatment can often be a combination of therapies. Patients with rectal cancer may have pre-operative radiotherapy or pre-operative chemo/radiotherapy followed by surgery while patients with malignant colonic tumours may go straight to surgery (Weiss & Johnson 1999).

Surgery may be either curative or palliative. If it is felt that the patient's cancer cannot be totally removed or if there are distant metastases (usually lung or liver) then palliative surgery may be carried out to relieve the patient's symptoms and prevent bowel obstruction. The patient may have to have a stoma formed, which can be either temporary or permanent.

Once diagnosed the cancer can only be truly staged following surgery when the histological specimen is examined. In the UK, this is done using either the modified Duke's or TNM classification.

Duke's grading (Weiss & Johnson 1999)

- Grade A – confined to mucosa.
- Grade B1 – involves part of muscle wall.
- Grade B2 – reaches the serosa.
- Grade C1 – involves wall, but not completely. Local lymph nodes involved.
- Grade C1 – involves serosa and lymph nodes.

TNM classification (Sonin & Wittekind 1997)

Primary tumour (T)

- TX – primary tumour cannot be assessed.
- T0 – no evidence of primary tumour.
- Ta – non-invasive papillary carcinoma.
- Tis – carcinoma *in situ*: 'flat tumour'.
- T1 – tumour invades subepithelial connective tissue.
- T2 – tumour invades muscle:
  - pT2a – tumour invades superficial muscle (inner half);
  - pT2b – tumour invades deep muscle (outer half).

- T3 – tumour invades perivesical tissue:
  - pT3a – microscopically;
  - pT3b – macroscopically (extravesical mass).
- T4 – tumour invades any of the following: prostate, uterus, vagina, pelvic wall, or abdominal wall:
  - T4a – tumour invades the prostate, uterus, vagina;
  - T4b – tumour invades the pelvic wall, abdominal wall.

Regional lymph nodes (N)

- NX – regional lymph nodes cannot be assessed.
- N0 – no regional lymph node metastasis.
- N1 – metastasis in a single lymph node, 2 cm or less in greatest dimension.
- N2 – metastasis in a single lymph node, more than 2 cm but not more than 5 cm in greatest dimension; or multiple lymph nodes, none more than 5 cm in greatest dimension.
- N3 – metastasis in a lymph node, more than 5 cm in greatest dimension.

Distant metastasis (M)

- MX – distant metastasis cannot be assessed.
- M0 – no distant metastasis.
- M1 – distant metastasis.

Abdominoperineal excision of rectum (APER)

APER is usually performed for carcinoma of the rectum. This major procedure can take between two and four hours and results in both a laparotomy and a perineal wound. The rectum, anal canal and sphincter muscles are removed necessitating formation of a permanent colostomy. Complications include poor perineal wound healing and urinary/sexual dysfunction. The use of stapling guns has allowed lower rectal anastomosis to be undertaken safely and consequently the number of patients having low anterior resections has

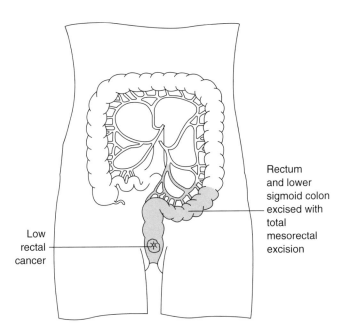

Low rectal cancer

Rectum and lower sigmoid colon excised with total mesorectal excision

Fig. 3.3 Abdominoperineal resection. Reproduced with kind permission of Aventis Pharma UK Ltd from Thomas, *A Guide to Colorectal Surgery*, 2001

increased with a subsequent drop in the number of patients requiring an APER (Nicholls 1996, Table 3.1; Fig. 3.3).

Anterior resection

Anterior resection involves removing part or all of the rectum and joining the sigmoid colon to the remaining rectum/anal canal. This procedure is commonly performed for cancer and may or may not result in a temporary loop ileostomy. If the cancer is situated in the upper (proximal) rectum, a temporary ileostomy is usually unnecessary as leak rates from the anastomosis are low (about 5%). If the cancer is situated in the lower (distal) rectum there is a higher risk of anastomotic leak

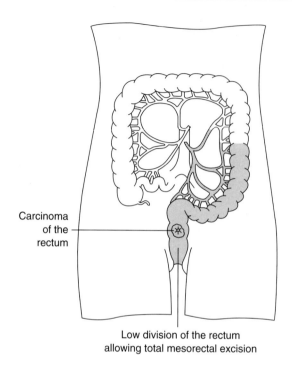

Carcinoma of the rectum

Low division of the rectum allowing total mesorectal excision

Fig. 3.4 Lower anterior resection of the rectum. Reproduced with kind permission of Aventis Pharma UK Ltd from Thomas, *A Guide to Colorectal Surgery*, 2001

(up to 30%) and therefore a temporary ileostomy is routinely used to protect the anastomosis until healing has occurred (Nicholls 1996, Table 3.1; Fig. 3.4).

TRAUMA

A variety of traumatic injuries may perforate the intestine and these include blunt trauma from road traffic accidents, shrapnel, and bullet and knife wounds. Unless the bowel is repaired the patients may develop peritonitis and die. According to

Steel *et al.* (2002) the recommended treatment for most traumatic colonic injuries is repair or resection and primary anastomosis. A temporary stoma is formed to allow healing to occur.

BOWEL ISCHAEMIA

If the blood supply to the bowel is compromised in any way necrosis will occur and this will lead to gangrene. The extent will depend on the vessels involved and the time that the bowel is starved of oxygen. Ischaemia is often caused by embolism or thrombosis in the mesentery. Most emboli originate from the heart (e.g. in patients with atrial fibrillation). Thrombosis usually occurs in patients with pre-existing stenosis of the mesenteric artery from atheroma (Goh 1997). Patients will require surgical intervention in which the necrotic segment is removed and a stoma is usually formed.

INCONTINENCE

Surgical intervention and stoma formation should only be considered when conservative methods have proved unsuccessful. However, if a patient's quality of life is suffering due to constant leakage of faecal matter alternative options will need to be considered. If the leakage is caused by damage to the anal sphincters the first possible surgical intervention should be to attempt to repair the anal sphincter, however, if this does not improve continence a stoma (end colostomy) may improve the patient's quality of life (see section on gracilis neosphincter in Chapter 2).

CARCINOMA OF THE BLADDER

The cause of bladder cancer is still unknown, although factors such as occupational exposure to carcinogens (such as rubber and dyes from the textile industry), smoking and the over-use of some analgesics are thought to play a part in its development (Blandy & Moors 1989). The disease affects four times as many men as women, and it is rare before the age of 50. The commonest form of the disease is *transitional cell carcinoma* (TCC). This is a cancer of the lining of the bladder and it is responsible for approximately 90% of all bladder cancers; 5–7% of bladder cancers are squamous carcinoma and 2–3% are adenocarcinomas. Bladder cancer (alongside prostate cancer) is the most common urological malignancy (Fenwick 1997).

Patients will usually present with haematuria (passing blood in the urine). A common investigation is cystoscopy – looking into the bladder with a fiber-optic telescope – this allows the bladder wall to be biopsied. Pathological staging of bladder cancer (Fenwick 1997):

- Tis – *in-situ* disease.
- Ta – epithelium only.
- T1 – lamina propria invasion.
- T2 – superficial muscle invasion.
- T3a – deep muscle invasion.
- T3b – perivesical fat invasion.
- T4 – prostate or contiguous muscle.

Treatment is dependent on staging of the tumour and a radical cystectomy is considered for patients who have T2–T3 tumours. This treatment is supplemented with both chemotherapy and radiotherapy.

Cystectomy

Cystectomy is usually performed for cancer. The bladder is removed and a 10–20 cm section of ileum is resected, but its blood supply maintained. The resected section of ileum has one end sutured closed and the ureters are anastomosed into it, the other end is brought to the surface of the abdominal wall as a urostomy (ileal conduit, see Chapter 2). The stoma is formed on the right side of the abdominal wall and the stoma is spouted like an ileostomy (Black 2000, Table 3.1; Fig. 3.5). Mitrofanoff pouch procedures are discussed in Chapter 2.

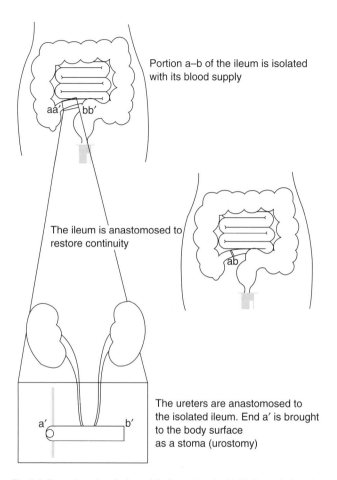

Portion a–b of the ileum is isolated with its blood supply

The ileum is anastomosed to restore continuity

The ureters are anastomosed to the isolated ileum. End a' is brought to the body surface as a stoma (urostomy)

Fig. 3.5 Formation of an ileal conduit. Reproduced with kind permission of Coloplast Ltd from *An Introduction to Stoma Care*, 2000

SELF-EVALUATION QUESTIONS AND ANSWERS

Questions

1. Which is the most common surgical procedure in a young person with fulminating colitis?
   A. Hartmann's procedure
   B. Koch pouch
   C. Ileo-anal pouch
   D. Total colectomy and formation of ileostomy

2. An abdominoperineal excision of rectum is commonly performed for:
   A. Faecal incontinence
   B. Rectal carcinoma
   C. Ulcerative colitis
   D. Crohn's disease

3. In a patient requiring emergency surgery for a perforated sigmoid diverticulum with faecal peritonitis, the most likely surgical procedure is:
   A. Low anterior resection
   B. Left hemicolectomy
   C. Hartmann's procedure
   D. Proctocolectomy

4. Panproctocolectomy results in which type of stoma?
   A. Double-barrel colostomy
   B. Loop ileostomy
   C. Kock continent ileostomy
   D. End ileostomy

5. In a patient with ulcerative colitis which systemic condition is not associated with ulcerative colitis:
   A. Ankylosing spondylitis
   B. Erythema nodosum
   C. Multiple colonic polyps
   D. Pyoderma gangrenosum

6. Which of the following statements is correct? Crohn's disease:
   A. Affects only the colon
   B. Can affect any part of the gastrointestinal tract from mouth to anus
   C. Affects the mucosa only
   D. Is treated primarily by surgery

Answers

1. D	4. D
2. B	5. C
3. C	6. B

REFERENCES

Afzal, M.A., Minor, F.D., Begley, J., Bentley, M.L., Armitage, E., Ghosh, S. & Ferguson, A. (1998) Absence of measles-virus genome in inflammatory bowel disease. *Lancet* **351**, 646–7.

Becker, J. (1999) Surgical therapy for ulcerative colitis and Crohn's disease. *Gastroenterology Clinics of North America* **28**, 371–89.

Black, P. (2000) In: *Holistic Stoma Care*. Ballière Tindall, London.

Blandy, J. & Moors, J. (1989) *Urology for Nurses*. Blackwell Science Publications, London.

Elcoat, C. (1986) Types of stoma and associated surgical procedures. In: C. Elcoat, ed. *Stoma Care Nursing – current nursing practice*. Baillière Tindall, London.

Farthing, M. (1993) Medical management of Crohn's disease and ulcerative colitis. In: C. Myers, ed. *Stoma Care Nursing: A Patient Centred Approach*, pp 42–62. Arnold, London.

Fenwick, E. (1997) Urological cancers. In: S. Fillingham & J. Douglas, eds. *Urological Nursing*. Balliere Tindall, London.

Forbes, A. (2002) Medical aspects of ulcerative colitis. In: J. Williams, ed. *The Essentials of Pouch Care Nursing*. Whurr Publishers, London.

Joels, J. (1999) Inflammatory bowel disease – the nursing implications. In: T. Porrett & N. Daniel, eds. *Essential Coloproctology for Nurses*. Whurr Publishers, London.

Goh, H. (1997) Intestinal ischaemia. In: R.T. Nicholls & R.R. Dozois, eds. *Surgery of the Colon and Rectum*. Churchill Livingstone, New York.

Hope, R.A., Longmore, J.M., Hodgetts, T.J. & Ramrakha, P.S. (1998) *Oxford Handbook of Clinical Medicine*, 4th edn. Oxford University Press, Oxford.

Kamm, M. (1996) *Inflammatory Bowel Disease*. Martin Dunitz, London.

Katz, J.A., Itoh, J. & Fiocchi, C. (1999) Pathogenesis of inflammatory bowel disease. *Current Opinion in Gastroenterology* **15**, 291.

Knowles, C. & Lunniss, P.J. (2003) Risk assessment and classification of septic diverticular disease. In: I. Taylor & C. Johnson, eds. *Recent Advances in Surgery*, Vol. 26. Royal Society of Medicine Press, London.

Neale, K. & Philips, R. (2002) Familial adenomatous polyposis. In: J. Williams, ed. *The Essentials of Pouch Care Nursing*. Whurr Publishers, London.

Nicholls, R.J. (1996) Surgical procedures. In: C. Myers, ed. *Stoma Care Nursing – A Patient Centred Approach*. Arnold, London.

Nogueras, J. & McGannon, E. (1999) Familial adenomatous polyposis. In: T. Porrett & N. Daniel, eds. *Essential Coloproctology for Nurses*. Whurr Publishers, London.

Peltola, H., Patja, A., Leinikki, P., Valle, M., Davidkin, I. & Paunio, M. (1998) No evidence for measles, mumps, and rubella vaccine-associated inflammatory bowel disease or autism in a 14-year prospective study. *Lancet* **351**, 1327–8.

Pullan, R. (1996) Colonic mucus, smoking and ulcerative colitis. *Annals of the Royal College of Surgeons of England* **78**, 85–91.

Sartor, P.B. (1993) Role of the intestinal microflora in pathogenesis and complications. In: J. Schölmerich, W. Kruis, H. Goebell, *et al.*, eds. *Inflammatory Bowel Diseases. Pathophysiology as Basis of Treatment*, pp. 175–87. Kluwer Academic Publishers, Germany.

Schoetz, D.J. (1993) Uncomplicated diverticulitis. In: B.G., Wolf, ed. *Surgical Clinics of North America*. WB Saunders, Philadelphia.

Sher, M.E., Cheney, L. & Ricciardi, J. (1999) Diverticular disease. In: T. Porrett & N. Daniel, eds. *Essential Coloproctology for Nurses*. Whurr Publishers, London.

Sonin, L.H. & Wittekind, C., eds. (1997) *TNM Classification of Malignant Tumours*, 5th edn, p. 227. John Wiley & Sons Inc., New York.

Stallmach, A. & Carstens, O. (2002) Role of infections in the manifestation or reactivation of inflammatory bowel diseases. *Inflammatory Bowel Diseases* **8**, 213–18.

Steel, M., Danne, P. & Jones, I. (2002) Colon trauma: Royal Melbourne Hospital experience. *New Zealand Journal of Surgery* **72**, 357.

Thompson, N.P. (1995) Is measles a risk for inflammatory bowel disease? *Lancet* **345**, 1071–3.

Turnburg, L. (1989) *Clinical Gastroenterology*. Blackwell Scientific, Oxford.

Weiss, E. & Johnson, T. (1999) Colorectal cancer. In: T. Porrett & N. Daniel, eds. *Essential Coloproctology for Nurses*, Whurr Publishers, London.

Wight, N. & Scott, B.B. (1997) Dietary treatment of active Crohn's disease. *British Medical Journal* **314**, 454–5.

Stoma Siting and the Role of the Clinical Nurse Specialist

4

Anthony McGrath & Patricia Black

INTRODUCTION

This chapter discusses the importance of stoma siting pre-operatively and the role of the clinical nurse specialist (CNS). The careful siting of a stoma pre-operatively, whether the stoma is to be permanent or temporary, plays an essential role in the rehabilitation of the patient (Black 2000). Reasons for the technique used and the consequences of incorrect siting will be examined.

LEARNING OBJECTIVES

By the end of the chapter the reader will be able to:

❏ understand who should site a stoma;
❏ understand the type and position of a colostomy, ileostomy and urostomy;
❏ understand the principles of stoma siting.

IMPORTANCE OF STOMA SITING

Before stoma therapists became part of the multidisciplinary team, the siting of a stoma was left to the surgeon and it was often decided after the patient was anaesthetised, and towards the end of the operation. Wade (1989), in her study of stoma therapists and their patients, found that even in trusts with stoma therapists, only a third of patients had their stoma sited by the stoma therapist. Although there appears to be no evidence base for stomas sited by stoma therapists being superior to those sited by a surgeon, there is a great probability that this will be the case (Padilla & Grant, 1985). The stoma therapist will have spent time with the patient, asked about lifestyle and clothing and have seen the patient in a variety of positions that will affect the stoma placing. The surgeon will have seen the patient in the hospital setting and in a different capacity and will probably not be aware of social impediments that may cause difficulty in siting a stoma (Black 2000). If a stoma therapist is not available the stoma may be sited by other qualified staff such as an experienced nurse who has had a training in stoma care or an experienced doctor (Bass *et al.*, 1997).

PATIENT ASSESSMENT

When assessing and discussing with the patient their impending stoma surgery it is important that the patient understands a basic outline of their gastrointestinal tract. The therapist should indicate the site of the stoma on a diagram. Involving the patient at all stages pre-operatively enables the patient to assimilate what can be devastating news and make informed choices about their care (Myers 1996).

When the stoma therapist first meets the patient, the nurse is mentally assessing the patient's physique – tall, short, fat, thin, male, female and any obvious physical disabilities. Lifestyle, leisure activities, sports and employment will be elicited from the patient. If the patient is employed, the nature of employment is important as heavy lifting, contact sport, labourers and those engaged in strenuous work and exercise may be prone to parastomal hernia or prolapsed stoma.

The importance of having a stoma correctly sited cannot be over-stressed and it is important that the nurse recognises that a minority of patients will not be western Caucasian but from other ethnic minorities, and religious and cultural influences will be important when the stoma is sited (CORCE 1997; Black 2004a). A patient's cultural and religious beliefs can have an effect on the choices they make about therapeutic interventions for stoma surgery and many will have specific beliefs about bodily excretions and consider them polluting and therefore not be willing to care for a stoma. In South Asian and Muslim cultures, traditionally the left hand is used for cleansing and hygiene and the right hand for eating and touching things. This may cause difficulty after stoma formation and the nurse needs to work with the patient pre-operatively to enable the patient to understand what will happen after surgery and how he or she will cope (Black 2000; Henley & Schott 2003; Black 2004b).

Fasting is often important for patients who are Hindus, Sikhs, Jews, Rastafarians and some Christians, but many Muslim patients may want to observe Ramadan when they do not eat or drink during the hours from sunrise to sunset (Black 1994; Cline 1995; Black 2004b). Also there may be issues as to where the stoma is placed on the abdomen and during the assessment stoma siting should be discussed with the patient. For a Caucasian patient, a stoma sited above the umbilicus would be difficult as the natural waistline is near the umbilicus. For a Muslim patient, a stoma sited below the umbilicus can cause distress as they would consider the output to be faeces, but sited above the umbilicus the output is considered to be food content and therefore acceptable (Black 1992; Black 2000; Kuzu *et al.* 2002).

ESSENTIAL INFORMATION FOR SITING A STOMA
When siting a stoma the stoma therapist or experienced person siting the stoma should have the following essential information.

- The type of surgery and stoma to be raised.
- Whether the patient has any obvious disabilities and uses straps or belts to support artificial limbs.
- Does the patient need glasses or hearing aid?
- Does the patient fully understand the primary language used?
- Can the patient give consent?

If the stoma is a colostomy it will be in the left iliac fossa and if the stoma is to be an ileostomy or urostomy it will be sited in the right iliac fossa.

SITING PROCEDURE

The nurse introduces him or herself to the patient and explains the procedure. The curtains are pulled around the bed and the patient is asked to expose the abdominal area between chest and groin. The patient is asked to lie on the bed with one pillow under the head and the arms by their side. Putting the arms behind the head while the nurse is talking to the patient pulls the abdomen into a higher position and leads to the incorrect siting of the stoma. With the patient lying flat examine the abdomen for signs of previous surgery, skin creases, hip bones, gullies, skin folds or skin problems such as psoriasis or eczema.

Areas to be avoided for a stoma site are:

- the waistline;
- hipbones;
- previous scar lines;
- groin areas;
- fat folds or bulges;
- umbilicus;
- current fistula or drain sites;
- under pendulous breasts;
- primary incision site;
- areas that have skin problems;
- areas crossed by straps for artificial limbs;
- areas where if there is weight loss or gain the stoma would be occluded.

Having examined the abdomen thoroughly the nurse locates the abdominus rectus muscle (see Fig. 4.1). This abdominal muscle forms the natural 'corset' of the abdomen and is the muscle that helps to lift the head from the pillow. It is located by stretching the nurse's thumb and forefinger across the

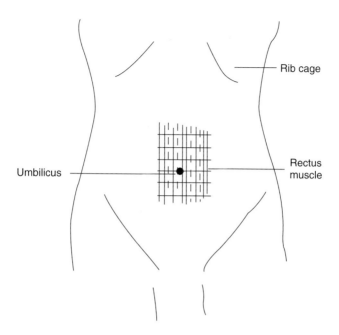

Fig. 4.1 Rectus muscle

middle of the abdomen just below the umbilicus and asking the patient to raise their head from the pillow. The muscle will be felt and often seen. Ideally, it is through this muscle that the stoma should be raised by the surgeon, having noticed the stoma therapist's mark (Black 2000).

The nurse makes a small mark at the appropriate site and side for either a colostomy, ileostomy or urostomy, being aware of the rectus abdominus muscle. The nurse then asks the patient first to sit up on the edge of the bed and then on a chair. While the patient is sitting on the bed and chair the nurse observes where the mark is. Do rolls of adipose tissue occlude it? Can the patient see the site? Will there be problems with waistlines of clothes? If the patient has their normal clothes with them it may help to try these on as well to see how the potential site is. If the patient is able to bend forwards towards their toes this will help to show how the stoma is placed. The patient can be offered an appropriate appliance to try over the site to see how it may affect their day-to-day activities and clothes (Black 2000).

Many older women become concerned that they will be unable to wear their support girdle or pants after stoma surgery. They can be reassured that support undergarments can be obtained on prescription once they have initially recovered from their surgery. This is not a prerogative of women; men may have support belts if needed, especially if their work is strenuous (Black 2000).

The nurse or stoma therapist must remember that a patient may gain a considerable amount of weight after surgery especially if they have suffered from inflammatory bowel disease, or the patient may lose weight if there is a diagnosis of cancer and this must be taken into account when siting a stoma.

Patients with disabilities, who spend most of their waking time in a wheelchair, should have the stoma sited while in the wheelchair. Suitable adjustments should be made to the siting of the stoma in conjunction and discussion with the patient.

When the appropriate site for the stoma has been agreed with the stoma therapist and patient, the nurse marks the site with a larger mark, such as a cross. This should be done with a dermatological skin marker as biro and felt-tip pens contain colophony, which may cause skin allergies. The mark should then be covered in a transparent sticky tape to prevent it being erased or washed off (Black 2000). It should be documented in the patient's medical and nursing notes that the site was marked in conjunction with the stoma therapist or nurse and with the patient's consent.

EMERGENCY SURGERY

Occasionally patients may arrive via the A&E department out of the hours of 9–5, and it may be deemed necessary that they have immediate surgery with the possibility of a stoma. If the bowel has perforated there may be peritonitis and the patient shocked and unable to assimilate much information (McGrath 1998). However today's guidelines for colorectal surgery (ACGBI 2001) recommend that if possible the patient be resuscitated and referred to the colorectal surgeons at the earliest moment to ensure appropriate surgery is undertaken and that there is a possibility of the stoma being sited by experienced staff.

Wade (1989) found that of patients who had undergone emergency stoma formation, 81.5% said they could see their stoma easily compared with 86.9% who had had elective surgery. In the elective cohort, 84.4% of stomas that were sited by the surgeon were visible to the patient, while 92% of those sited by the stoma therapist were easily visible to the patient. Wade's study and work by Bekkers *et al.* (1995, 1996) show that there is great importance attached to the correct siting of the stoma, and although the percentages do not show significant differences, for individual patients, who will have to cope for the rest of their lives, the differences are significant.

SELF-EVALUATION QUESTIONS AND ANSWERS

Questions

1. Who should site a stoma pre-operatively?
   A. The healthcare assistant
   B. The house officer
   C. The stoma therapist
   D. The ward clerk

2. Why is it important to know if the patient does heavy lifting or strenuous exercise?
   A. So that the nurse can arrange someone to help them
   B. There may be a risk of a parastomal hernia
   C. The patient may have indigestion
   D. The patient may have to change their employment

3. In which cultures is the left hand traditionally used for cleansing?
   A. Australian
   B. Caucasian
   C. South Asian and Muslim
   D. American

4. What should the stoma therapist know when siting the patient?
   A. The patient's age
   B. The patient's first name
   C. The type of stoma to be raised
   D. Whether the patient has any children

5. Where should the stoma not be sited?
   A. Below the umbilicus
   B. Right iliac fossa
   C. Left iliac fossa
   D. The primary incision site

6. Where should a stoma be sited?
   A. The rectus abdominus muscle
   B. The psoas muscle

7. How should a person with disabilities be sited for a stoma?
   A. Lying on the bed
   B. In their wheelchair

8. What will be the consequences for the patient with a stoma sited in the wrong place?

9. Name five religions where fasting plays an important role in the patient's life.

10. What essential information should a nurse be aware of when siting a stoma?

Answers

   1. C
   2. B
   3. C
   4. C
   5. D

6. A
7. B
8. Unable to manage their own self-care
9. Hinduism, Sikhism, Judaism, Rastafarian faith, Islam
10. • The type of stoma to be raised
    • Whether the patient has any disabilities that may cause an impediment
    • Whether the patient wears glasses or hearing aid
    • Does the patient understand the primary language used?
    • Can the patient give consent?

REFERENCES

Association of Coloproctology of Great Britain and Ireland (ACGBI) (2001) *Resources for Coloproctology.* ACGBI, London.

Bass, E.M., Pino, A., Tan, A., Pearl, R.K., Orsay, C.P. & Abcarian, H. (1997) Does preoperative stoma marking and education by the enterostomal therapist affect outcome? *Diseases of the Colon and Rectum* **40**, 440–2.

Bekkers, M., van Knippenberg, E., van den Borne, H., van Berge-Henegouwen, G., Poen, H. & Bergsma, J. (1995) Psychosocial adaptation to stoma surgery: a review. *Journal of Behavioural Medicine* **18**, 1–31.

Bekkers, M., van Knippenberg, E., van den Borne, H. & van Berge-Henegouwen, G. (1996) Prospective evaluation of psychosocial adaptation to stoma surgery: the role of self efficacy. *Psychosomatic Medicine* **58**, 183–91.

Black, P. (1992) Body image after enterostomal surgery. [Unpublished MSc thesis] Steinberg Collection. Royal College of Nursing, London.

Black, P. (1994) Hidden problems of stoma care. *British Journal of Nursing* **3**, 707–11.

Black, P. (2000) *Holistic Stoma Care.* Ballière Tindall, London.

Black, P. (2004a) The importance of palliative care for patients with colorectal cancer. *British Journal of Nursing* **13**, 584–9.

Black, P. (2004b) Psychological, sexual and cultural issues for patients with a stoma. *British Journal of Nursing* **13**, 692–7.

Cline, S. (1995) *Lifting the Taboo; Women, Death and Dying.* Little Brown & Co., London.

ConvaTec Ostomy Research Centre. (CORCE) (1997) *Stoma Siting.* Medical Projects International, Maidenhead.

Henley, A. & Schott, J. (2003) *Culture, Religion and Patient Care in a Multi-Ethnic Society.* Age Concern, London.

Kuzu, M., Ayhan, T., Omer, U., Keriman, U., Suat, U., Ekrem, E., *et al.* (2002) Effect of sphincter sacrificing surgery for rectal carcinoma on quality of life in Muslim patients. *Diseases of the Colon and Rectum* **45**, 1359–66.

McGrath, A. (1998) Abdominal assessment in A&E. *Emergency Nurse* **6**, 15–19.

Myers, C., ed. (1996) *Stoma Care Nursing – A Patient Centred Approach.* Arnold, London.

Padilla, G. & Grant, M. (1985) Quality of life as a cancer nursing outcome variable. *Advances in Nursing Science* **8**, 45–60.

Wade, B. (1989) *A Stoma is for Life.* Scutari Press, Harrow.

The Immediate Postoperative Period

Theresa Porrett

5

INTRODUCTION

In the pre-operative period the focus of nursing care will have been on the psychological preparation of the patient about to undergo stoma forming surgery. In the immediate postoperative period the physical support of the patient becomes the priority. During this initial postoperative period (one to five days) the patient is unable to care for the stoma (due to lack of knowledge and because they are recovering from surgery), and, therefore, the responsibility lies with the nurse. Once the patient begins to recuperate from surgery they can be involved in caring for their stoma and teaching can take place.

In addition to the routine postoperative observations required following any major abdominal surgery (vital signs, drains, pain control, fluid balance) specific observation and monitoring is required following stoma formation. A healthy stoma should be pink/red in colour (very similar to the colour of the mucosa in the mouth). To facilitate stomal observation, a newly formed stoma will be covered by a large transparent appliance, which does not have a flatus filter. These postoperative appliances are drainable as stomal output initially may be liquid in nature and may drain in large amounts (in an ileostomy over 1 l in 24 hours is not unusual).

The aim of this chapter is to outline the role of the nurse in the support and monitoring of patients immediately following stoma-forming surgery.

LEARNING OBJECTIVES
By the end of this chapter the reader will be able to:

❏ describe the monitoring of a stoma immediately following surgery;
❏ outline the potential postoperative stomal complications;
❏ describe the assessment of stomal function.

There are a number of postoperative management issues which are not specifically related to stoma formation, but all aspects of the postoperative period are covered below. The specific issues relating to a newly formed stoma and the potential stomal complications are outlined in Table 5.1 in the format of a nursing care plan.

ABDOMINAL WOUND DRESSING
The majority of patients who have undergone stoma forming surgery will have a midline laparotomy incision. It is usual for this wound to be dressed in theatres. The stoma appliance should be positioned securely first and then the wound dressing applied. This ensures that the appliance can adhere directly to the skin and not onto the wound dressing as this weakens the adhesion of the appliance and may cause the appliance to leak. The wound dressing will require changing if soiled, the dressing should never be placed under the stoma appliance as this will form an inadequate seal and leakage may result.

STOMAL ROD/BRIDGE
A rod or bridge is a specifically manufactured plastic rod which is used to support a loop stoma. The rod is positioned under the loop of bowel on top of the skin and prevents the loop from retracting into the abdominal cavity (see Plate 6). It usually remains in place for three to five days and is removed on the surgeon's instructions. One end of the rod has a swivel attachment, which can be straightened to allow the rod to be removed. This is a painless procedure but does require the appliance to be removed and replaced with a new appliance

Table 5.1 Postoperative care plan outlining potential stoma problems

Potential problem	Action	Rationale/evidence
Ischaemia or necrosis of the stoma	• Transparent appliance in place	• Occurs in 23% of newly formed stomas (Lyon & Smith 2001)
• Most common during the first 48 hours postoperatively	• Observe the stoma every four hours and note its colour and size.	• Can be caused by local oedema and occlusion of the blood supply by a tight fitting appliance
• Caused by inadequate blood supply to the stoma (Erwin-Toth & Doughty 1992; McCahon 1999)	• The stoma should be pink. If colour darkens to purple/black ischaemia may be present	• If superficial ischaemia the tissue will 'slough' off and the stoma will function normally
• The stoma appears dry, firm to the touch, may feel cool and the colour is dark red, purplish or black (Bradley 1997)	• Report immediately to nurse in charge/surgeon	• Early detection allows review and change of appliance and may prevent surgical intervention being required
• The ischaemia or necrosis may be superficial and result in sloughing off of the tissue; if deep, surgical revision will be required (Lee 2001)		
• See Plate 1		

Contd

Table 5.1 *Continued*

Potential problem	Action	Rationale/evidence
Paralytic ileus • This is the absence of bowel sounds and failure to pass flatus	• The time when the stoma first acts and the quantity of the output should be noted and recorded on the fluid balance chart (Coloplast 1995)	• This information is important as it indicates that peristalsis has re-started and will influence when the patient may commence on oral fluids
• Normal response to surgical manipulation and bowel anaesthesia	• First passage of flatus also should be noted (the appliance does not have a filter so will distend with flatus) (Coloplast 1995)	
• Usually resolves after 48–72 hours (Erwin-Toth & Doughty 1992)		
High output from stoma • This may cause electrolyte imbalance and appliance leakage	• Most common in first two to seven days after surgery in ileostomists	• If an ileostomy has been formed, the patient has lost the major salt and water reabsorbing organ of the body and is at risk of profound disturbances in electrolyte balance (Coloplast 1995)

Mucocutaneous separation

- This is the breakdown of the suture line securing the stoma to the abdominal surface (Erwin-Toth & Doughty 1992; Bradley 1997; Collett 2002)
- It may affect the whole suture line or just part of it
- See Plate 2

- Accurate measurement and recording of fluid intake and output
- Record stomal output on fluid balance chart

- Observe the stoma during routine appliance change and note position of sutures around stoma
- Report any signs of mucocutaneous separation to the stoma care nurse specialist (SCN)
- Apply hydrocolloid paste (Stomahesive or Granuflex paste) to the area as recommended by the SCN

- If output from stoma is over 1 l the patient may require fluid/electrolyte replacement to prevent dehydration
- The weight of the filled appliance may compromise adhesion of the flange and cause leakage problems (Elcoat 1986)

- May cause stomal retraction or stenosis so observation and reporting to SCN essential to ensure long-term follow-up of the patient

- If superficial is managed by the SCN

- If deep may require surgical intervention to re-suture the stoma

Contd

Table 5.1 *Continued*

Potential problem	Action	Rationale/evidence
Flushed or retracted stoma		
• The stoma is pulled back into the abdominal cavity and does not protrude above the level of the skin (McCahon 1999; Myers 1996)	• Observe stoma through clear appliance or during routine appliance change and report any change in protrusion of stoma	
• It is caused by the bowel being under tension, usually due to inadequate bowel mobilisation at operation or in obese patients (Collett 2002)	• To prevent leakage, pastes, seals or convexity might be required to create an adequate seal. The SCN will advise on the use of these products (and which is most suitable)	
• See Plate 3		
Skin excoriation (effluent dermatitis)		
• This is not uncommon in the initial postoperative period, especially if a stomal rod has been in place (Arumugam *et al.* 2002)	• Observe peri-stomal skin during routine appliance change and report any skin discoloration to the SCN	
• Caused by leakage of stomal effluent onto the peri-stomal skin	• Apply skin barrier cream as advised by the SCN	

- See Plate 4

Oedema

- This is not uncommon in the first one to seven days postoperatively

- The stoma can appear taut and shiny (Bradley 1997)

- See Plate 5

- Ensure aperture in flange is cut to the correct size, ensuring no peri-stomal skin is left exposed

- Observe

- If the stoma becomes oedematous the flange aperture will need to be increased in size

- When the oedema resolves the aperture in the flange will need to be made smaller to ensure all peri-stomal skin is protected

- The stoma can reduce in size postoperatively up to 30% (Cottam 1998) but this can take up to eight weeks (Collett 2002)

- The SCN will teach the patient how to check the appliance template and resize it to accommodate this shrinkage in size afterwards. It is normally undertaken by the stoma care nurse (SCN), as once removed patients can usually start using an opaque smaller drainable or closed appliance.

SUTURES

Stitches or staples may be used to close the laparotomy wound. These are removed around ten days postoperatively, on the surgeon's instructions. There will be sutures around the mucocutaneous border of the stoma. These are always dissolvable sutures and do not need to be removed. They can take from one to three weeks to dissolve and patients need to be informed that when cleaning and drying the stoma they may notice the sutures coming away on the wipe they are using.

URETERIC STENTS

One of the main differences in the postoperative management of a patient having undergone urostomy formation is the presence of urinary stents (see Plate 7). These fine-bore stents are placed in the ureters at the point of the anastomosis (joining with the small bowel). They prevent urinary leakage from the anastomosis and ensure the ureters remain patent (Black 2000). (The ureters can become oedematous immediately after surgery and may prevent urinary flow from the kidney.) These stents usually remain in place for seven to ten days and are removed before the patient is discharged home. The SCN will normally remove the stents. When changing an appliance the stents must be passed through the opening in the flange and down into the pouch.

GENERAL HYGIENE

Once mobile a patient may bath or shower. Until the abdominal wound has healed this should be done with the stoma appliance in place. Once the abdominal wound has healed patients may bath or shower without the appliance in place, drying the peri-stomal skin and applying a new appliance once they have completed their bathing.

NUTRITION

For the first few days following bowel surgery the patient will take nothing orally and will have their fluid requirements administered via an intravenous infusion. This regimen continues until bowel sounds are heard or the patient passes flatus into the stoma appliance. Oral fluids are commenced by generally starting at 30–60 ml an hour (water) until the patient is tolerating these fluids with no nausea/vomiting. If a nasogastric tube is in place it will be spigotted once the patient commences oral fluids. Once tolerating free fluids patients will commence a light diet.

CHANGING THE POST-OPERATIVE APPLIANCE IN THE FIRST 24–72 HOURS

The SCN will have left supplies of the correct postoperative appliance, these will usually be in the patient's locker. Do not change the postoperative appliance routinely, these appliances can remain in place for up to five days. Change the appliance only if requested to do so by the SCN, if there is leakage from the stoma or if closer observation of the stoma and peri-stomal skin is required.

Follow the guidelines given in Chapter 9 to change the appliance. It is important to remember the following points:

- The abdomen may be bruised and tender following surgery.
- The procedure may be painful so be as gentle as possible.
- The patient may not wish to look at the stoma at this early stage.
- The patient will potentially be very sensitive about the stoma and will be acutely aware of any facial signs of disgust on your face. Ensure you do not react negatively (verbally or facially) when changing the appliance as this will reinforce the patient's feelings of unacceptability and will hinder their psychological adaptation (Ewing 1989).
- Patients will be very aware of odour from the stoma both during emptying and changing of the appliance. Use a

deodorising spray after the procedure to ensure no residual odours are left.

SELF-EVALUATION QUESTIONS AND ANSWERS

Questions

Mr Jones is a 72-year-old gentleman who had elective surgery for a low rectal carcinoma. He had an abdominal perineal excision of rectum and formation of an end colostomy. A clear one-piece drainable appliance was applied in theatre.

1. What is the purpose of this specific type of appliance?
2. Why are flatus filters not used during the initial postoperative period when the patient is nil by mouth?

Mr Jones has been back on the ward for 2 hours when you observe that the stoma has become slightly larger in size and is a darker red colour than when you last observed it.

3. What might be the cause of this increase in stomal size?

Miss Jacobs, a 54-year-old obese lady, is recovering from surgery to remove her bladder. Three days previously she underwent a total cystectomy and formation of urostomy. Miss Jacobs complains of feeling liquid on her abdomen and when you check the appliance you note that it is leaking urine from under the flange. You prepare to change the appliance and on removing the leaking appliance you notice that there is mucocutaneous separation.

4. What would you do on noticing the mucocutaneous seperation?

5. How might this be treated?

6. At what stage of a patient's recovery is the rod usually removed from a loop stoma?

7. What factors may cause ischaemia or necrosis of the stoma?

Answers

1. A clear appliance is used in the immediate postoperative period to allow observation of the colour and size of the stoma. The appliance is drainable to ensure that any haemoserous fluid, bile or faecal fluid can be emptied when necessary. The appliance has a long-lasting adhesive, which means the appliance can be left in place for up to five days.

2. Filters are not routinely inserted in postoperative appliances as it is important to be able to note when the patient begins passing flatus, this is a sign that paralytic ileus is resolving.

3. Postoperative oedema. It is normal for the stoma to be slightly bruised and swollen initially after surgery due to the manual handling of the bowel during the operation.

4. Inform the SCN. If the mucocutanous separation is superficial it can be conservatively managed.

5. Often a hydrocolloid paste such as Stomahesive paste can be used to fill in the skin defect aound the stoma caused by the mucocutaneous separation. If left unfilled urine can collect in the skin defect and cause leakage. If the defect is deeper Granuflex paste may be used to promote wound healing and also prevent leakage. Once applied into the skin defect the area is covered as normal by the adhesive flange of the appliance.

6. The rod usually remains in place for three to five days and is removed on the surgeon's instructions. Removal prematurely could lead to stomal retraction.

7. Ischaemia/necrosis is caused by an inadequate blood supply to the stoma, this is usually a result of the surgery but it may be caused by stomal oedema or occlusion of the blood supply by a tight-fitting appliance.

REFERENCES

Arumugam, P.J., Bevan, L., Macdonald, L., Watkins, A., Morgan, A., Beynon, J. *et al.* (2002) A prospective audit of stomas – analysis of risk factors and complications and their management. *Colorectal Disease* **5**, 49–52.

Black, P. (2000) *Holistic Stoma Care.* Ballière Tindall, London.

Bradley, M. (1997) Essential elements of ostomy care. *American Journal of Nursing* **97**, 38–45.

Collett, K. (2002) Practical aspects of stoma management. *Nursing Standard* **17**, 45–52.

Coloplast, Ltd. (1995) *Ostomy and Ostomy Patients – An Introductory Guide for Nurses.* Coloplast, Peterborough.

Cottam, J. (1998) Bowel stomas: coping with a problem. *Charter* **4**, 12–13. Coloplast, Peterborough.

Elcoat, C. (1986) Postoperative stoma care. In: E. Elcoat, ed. *Stoma Care Nursing.* Ballière Tindall, London.

Erwin-Toth, P. & Doughty, D. (1992) Principles and procedures of stomal management. In: B. Hampton & R. Bryan, eds. *Ostomies and Continent Diversions – Nursing Management.* Mosby Year Book, St Louis.

Ewing, G. (1989) The nursing preparation of stoma patients for self-care. *Journal of Advanced Nursing* **14**: 411–20.

Lee, J. (2001) Common stoma problems: a brief guide for community nurses. *British Journal of Community Nursing* **6**, 407–13.

Lyon, C. & Smith, A. (2001) *Abdominal Stomas and Their Skin Disorders – An Atlas of Diagnosis and Management.* Martin Dunitz, London.

McCahon, S. (1999) Faecal stomas. In T. Porrett & N. Daniel, eds. *Essential Coloproctology for Nurses.* Whurr Publishers, London.

Myers, C. (1996) Appliance leakage. In: C. Myers, ed. *Stoma Care Nursing – A Patient Centred Approach.* Arnold, London.

Choosing the Correct Stoma Appliance

6

Jude Cottam & Theresa Porrett

INTRODUCTION

Patients undergoing stoma surgery will adapt to their new body image and integrate back into their social circle more readily if they receive empathic input from the pre-operative period through to their return into the community (Black 2000). Using the correct appliance is a major contributing factor to the physical and psychological well-being of the patient. Advances in technology and the millions of pounds spent by manufacturers in product development has revolutionised the range and choice of appliances now available to patients (Black 2000).

Today's appliances bear no resemblance to those of days gone by when pouches were made out of rubber and changing a bag was almost a 'surgical procedure'. Nowadays, appliances include hypoallergenic adhesives and protective covers to avoid skin irritation (Black 2000). The effluent from a stoma can damage unprotected skin, ileostomists are particularly at risk due to the high enzyme content of the output (Dyer 1988).

LEARNING OBJECTIVES

By the end of this chapter the reader will be able to:

❏ describe the different types of stoma appliances;
❏ identify the correct type of appliance for an ileostomy, colostomy and urostomy;
❏ give the rationale for choice of one- or two-piece appliance;
❏ give the rationale for the choice of closed or drainable appliance.

Stoma care equipment is available in various shapes and guises, the type used being dependent on a number of individual patient factors:

- type of stoma and its output;
- site of stoma;
- skin sensitivity;
- stage of rehabilitation of the patient;
- patient's cognitive and motor skills;
- patient's lifestyle.

There are four main categories of appliance:

- one-piece appliance (Fig. 6.1);
- two-piece appliance (Fig. 6.2);
- clear appliance (Figs 6.1 & 6.2);
- opaque appliance (Figs 6.1 & 6.2).

ONE-PIECE APPLIANCE

This is an appliance, which following removal of the backing paper from the adhesive barrier ring, is placed over the stoma adhering directly onto the skin. This means the appliance and

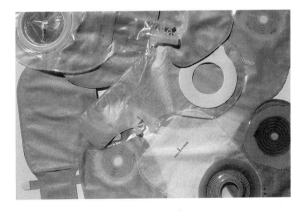

Fig. 6.1 Range of one-piece appliances, clear and opaque

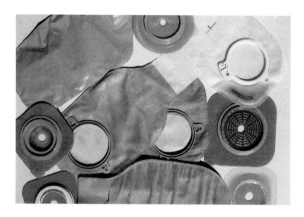

Fig. 6.2 Range of two-piece appliances, clear and opaque

adhesive flange are sealed together (see Fig. 6.1). A one-piece appliance may have a pre-cut opening, which should fit neatly around the stoma, protecting the surrounding skin, or the opening may need to be cut to the correct size of the stoma particularly if it is irregular in shape (Dyer 1988). The complete appliance is discarded once it is removed and replaced as necessary. A patient needs to be dexterous and well motivated to manage this type of pouch. These appliances tend to be soft and flexible and are discreet under clothing.

TWO-PIECE APPLIANCE

A two-piece appliance consists of a base plate (flange) of skin-protective and adhesive material and a pouch (see Fig. 6.2). Following the cutting of the flange to the size of the stoma and removal of the backing paper, the flange is placed over the stoma adhering directly onto the skin. The pouch is then clipped to the flange (Dyer 1988).

The advantage of this type of system is that the bag can be changed without removing the flange from the skin and therefore this causes less trauma to the skin. This type of appliance is useful for those patients who are less dexterous and/or partially sighted. Partially sighted patients can benefit from being able to attach the bag to the flange by touch, and are therefore able to independently manage the stoma often only requiring the district nurse to visit every four to five days to change the flange. The disadvantage of this type of appliance is that it tends to be more rigid against the abdomen and because of the plastic ring on the bag and flange (the attaching mechanism) it is less discreet under clothing.

CLEAR APPLIANCE

A clear appliance is recommended for a minimum of 48 hours following surgery to enable the stoma colour and output to be observed and monitored.

A clear appliance can be useful when the patient is being taught stoma management as it allows the patient to see that the appliance has been correctly positioned over the stoma (see Figs 6.1 & 6.2). For this reason it is often used by those patients who are partially sighted. A urostomist may wish to monitor the colour of their urine to ensure the urine is not too concentrated and therefore a clear appliance is often used.

OPAQUE APPLIANCE

An opaque appliance is preferred by many patients for aesthetic reasons. The opaque material and synthetic cover masks the faeces or urine from view (see Figs 6.1 & 6.2). These days the synthetic covers are flesh coloured and almost resemble underwear, which has a positive impact on the patient's body image.

All the four main appliance categories outlined above also come in a range of closed and drainable forms.

DRAINABLE APPLIANCE

A drainable appliance has an open end which is sealed with a clip (see Figs 6.1 & 6.2). This is to enable the contents to be drained as necessary. These pouches are suitable for stomas which produce semi-formed or liquid faeces, e.g. in the postoperative period, right transverse colostomy, ileostomy and the management of fistulae or wound drains. Most drainable appliances also have a charcoal-based integrated filter, which allows flatus to be released but without odour. The frequency of change can vary from daily to every three to four days.

The urostomy appliance has a non-return valve inside to prevent urine flowing back over the skin and stoma (Black 1994) and a drainage tap at the bottom, which can be attached to a drainage bag at night (see Figs 6.1 & 6.2).

CLOSED APPLIANCE

Closed appliances have no opening other than the aperture to fit over the stoma. There is a charcoal-based integrated filter, which allows flatus to be released odour free. This appliance is suitable for left-sided transverse and sigmoid colostomies and is changed once or twice a day. If a two-piece appliance is in use, then the recommended wear time for the flange is five to seven days.

As with all guidelines (Table 6.1) there are exceptions to the standard appliance choice (Table 6.2). For example, an ileostomist with poor manual dexterity or diminished eyesight may manage and be self-caring or independent with a

Table 6.1 Types of stoma and the appropriate appliance to use

Type of stoma	Output	Type of pouch	Wear time
Colostomy	Formed/semi-formed	Closed	12–24 hours
Transverse colostomy	Semi-formed/liquid	Closed or drainable	12–72 hours
Ileostomy	Semi-formed/liquid	Drainable	12–72 hours
Urostomy	Urine	Drainable	24–72 hours

Table 6.2 Exceptions to the standard appliance choice

Type of stoma	Output	Type of pouch	Rationale
Colostomy	Diarrhoea	Drainable	If using a one-piece – will avoid trauma to the skin due to frequent removal of pouch, e.g. following the administration of bowel preparation for colonoscopy If using a two-piece – will be more cost effective
Ileostomy	>1000 ml	Drainable attached to free drainage	Will avoid overfilling of the pouch with subsequent leakage and facilitate the measurement of output to maintain accurate fluid balance

two-piece closed rather than a drainable appliance, which they may have problems emptying. Although the patient will be guided and advised by the stoma care specialist nurse, ultimately the type of appliance used is the patient's choice.

If an established stoma patient is an emergency admission to your ward area and does not have their stoma care equipment with them, it is important to focus on the type rather than the make of the pouch, i.e. closed or drainable rather than the manufacturer. Table 6.3 outlines the assessment you would undertake prior to advising or supplying a patient with a stoma appliance.

The manufacturers of stoma care appliances together with SCNs are continually striving to develop the ultimate appliance to provide the patient with the optimum quality of life (Black 1995). Consequently, new appliances are constantly becoming available. The SCN is best placed to advise patients on new product developments which may be suitable for them.

Table 6.3 Appliance Assessment Guidelines. Reproduced with permission from the Royal College of Nursing *Principle – A framework of nursing designed specifically for meeting the needs of stoma care patients 1994*

Assessment	Problem	Goal	Action
Physique	Stature Weight Contours	Appliance to be comfortable and mould to body contours	Ostomy pouches available in a range of lengths and shape, e.g. standard, small, mini Flange soft and flexible or rigid and convex
Mental ability	Age Intelligence	Simplicity	Acquisition of new skills can be difficult
Physical ability and manual dexterity	Disability, e.g. paraplegia Capability, e.g. arthritis	Promote patient's independence	May need assistance with stoma care Consider pre-cut apertures
Shape, size and site of stoma	Badly sited stoma Irregular shape Large/small	Appliance security Appliance to fit snugly around base of stoma	Ensure a flat surface for appliance adhesion Appliances with a starter hole will adapt to shape of stoma Measure stoma correctly using a guide or template. Allow 3 mm clearance

Contd

Table 6.3 *Continued*

Assessment	Problem	Goal	Action
Skin	Previous skin condition, e.g. eczema Sensitive skin	Minimise trauma Maintain security and dignity	Patch test prior to surgery Hypoallergenic adhesive Two-piece appliance incorporating skin protective wafer Skin care aids, e.g. lotions, barrier films
Type of stoma	Consistency of effluent, soft, firm, liquid Frequency of action Flatus	Knowledge and understanding of surgery	Closed end appliance less than two pouches daily or two-piece system Drainable open-ended device May require dietary advice or medication to regulate bowel action Consider pouch with activated charcoal filter
Lifestyle	Mobility Social Financial Individual needs	Pre-operative siting of stoma, to minimise interference with lifestyle Promote rehabilitation	Range of appliances available to enable needs of the individual to be met Ensure patient awareness of prescription exemption if permanent stoma Discuss other forms of management, e.g. irrigation, plug systems if appropriate

SELF-EVALUATION QUESTIONS AND ANSWERS

Questions

1. Mrs Brown has had a colostomy for three years and has been admitted to your ward for a colonoscopy. She is currently using a one-piece closed pouch. She has had a colonoscopy before and is worried that she will make her skin sore by frequent changing of the pouch when the bowel preparation begins to work as this is what happened the last time. What options can you give her to prevent this?

2. Mr Jones has a urostomy which over-fills at night causing a wet bed. He is currently using a one-piece drainable pouch with a tap and has tried attaching to a night drainage system but the pouch twisted and subsequently leaked. What advice can you give him?

3. Mrs Smith has a transverse colostomy sited in the right upper quadrant which she has had for three months. She uses a one-piece drainable pouch which she was draining three to four times a day. For the last two weeks the output has been less from the colostomy, needing attention only twice a day. The consistency is now semi-formed and she is finding it difficult and unpleasant to remove from the pouch. What are her appliance options?

Answers

1. There are two potential options for Mrs Brown:

   Option 1 – a one-piece drainable pouch to allow the faecal fluid to be drained away as needed.

   Option 2 – a two-piece closed system, this allows the flange to remain in place and the pouch is changed only when necessary.

2. A two-piece system would allow Mr Jones to remove the pouch and place it at the correct angle to facilitate the flow of urine without disturbing his skin.

3. There are two potential options for Mrs Smith:

   Option 1 – a one-piece closed pouch, which will be changed twice a day

   Option 2 – a two-piece closed system. The flange stays in place for three to five days and the pouch is removed as needed.

REFERENCES

Black, P. (1994) Choosing the correct stoma appliance. *British Journal of Nursing* **3**, 545–50.

Black, P. (1995) Stoma care: finding the most appropriate appliance. *British Journal of Nursing* **4**, 188–92.

Black, P. (2000) Practical stoma care. *Nursing Standard* **14**, 47–53.

Dyer, S. (1988) Stoma care: choosing the right appliance. *Professional Nurse* **3**, 278–82.

Royal College of Nursing (1994) *Principle – A Framework of Nursing Designed Specifically for Meeting the Needs of Stoma Patients*, RCN, London.

Accessories Used in Stoma Care

7

Anthony McGrath & Antoinette Johnson

INTRODUCTION

There are numerous problems that can affect those with a temporary or permanent stoma. Stoma problems can occur immediately postoperatively, during hospitalisation or after discharge (Collett 2002). These problems are categorised into physiological, psychological and physical complications (Lawson 2003). Following stoma formation about 39% of colostomy patients and 55% of ileostomy and urostomy patients will experience problems with stoma management (Lyon & Smith 2001).

This chapter aims to discuss the physical problems of a stoma that can occur after discharge from hospital and their practical management with the use of stoma care accessories.

LEARNING OBJECTIVES

By the end of this chapter the reader will be:

❏ able to recognise various physical problems of a stoma;
❏ aware of the stoma care accessory products that are available;
❏ able to provide possible solutions to physical problems of a stoma.

STOMA PROBLEMS

Most stoma problems are seen in the first year after surgery (Wade 1989). The incidence of stoma problems with new stomas has been estimated to range from 3% to 38% (Breeze 2000). Problems with established stomas become more evident later; this is usually due to a change in lifestyle or occupation. Stoma problems can be managed by educating patients and making certain changes in their stoma management with the use of stoma care accessories. The various stoma problems and solutions are discussed below.

Herniation can occur around the stoma; it is called a parastomal hernia. It is more common in end colostomies and occurs in 20–24% of cases (Devlin 1982). It is more prevalent in the older age group due to diminished muscle tone. The degree of a parastomal hernia can vary from a slight bulge to a large hernia with the stoma at the apex or retracted beneath the hernia bulge. The reasons a parastomal hernia might develop include the positioning of the stoma outside the rectus muscle, the aperture through the abdominal wall being large at the time of surgery, multiple surgical procedures and heavy lifting. Surgical repair will only be necessary in extreme cases and there is still a risk of hernia formation at the new site. Conservative management with the use of an abdominal support belt and educating the patient is usually sufficient to alleviate this problem.

Effluent dermatitis is characterised by inflamed excoriated and weeping skin caused by the leakage of effluent on to it. It is estimated that approximately 19% of patients will suffer from this problem (Borwell 1996). The reasons for effluent leaking on to the skin can be due to negligence in personal hygiene, diminished eye sight and a lack of manual dexterity. Incorrect appliance fitting, a too large pouch aperture in relation to stoma size or creases/dips around the stoma leading to leakage onto the skin are all possible causes (see also Table 5.1).

Careful assessment to identify the cause and to establish the appropriate stoma care accessory needed to resolve the problem is essential. The sore skin needs to be protected from the effluent which can be achieved by using barrier sprays, wipes or creams or protective powders applied to the skin. Pastes or adhesive seals can be used in filling the peristomal creases/dips. Selecting an alternative appliance, correct sizing

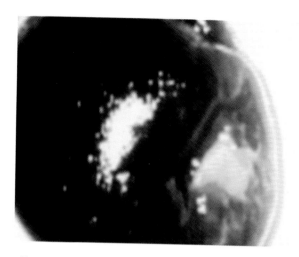

Plate 1 Necrotic stoma. Reproduced with permission.

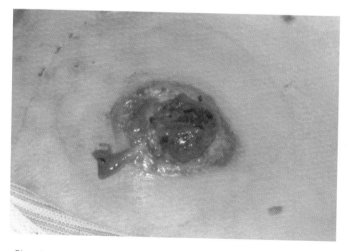

Plate 2 Mucocutaneous separation. Reproduced with permission

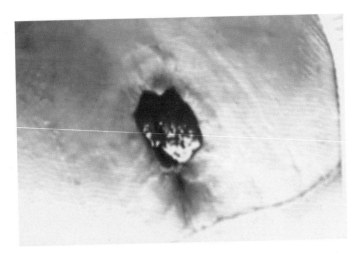

Plate 3 Retracted stoma. Reproduced with permission

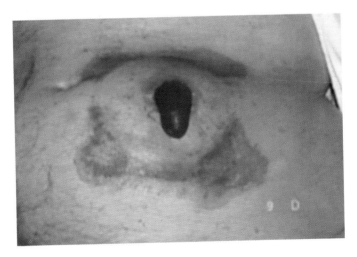

Plate 4 Skin excoriation. Reproduced with permission

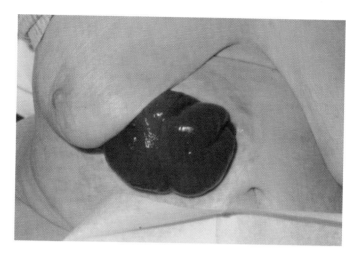

Plate 5 Oedematous stoma. Reproduced with permission

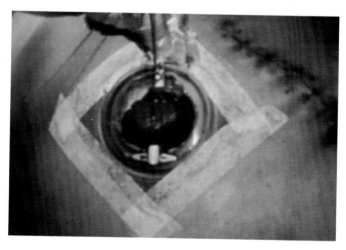

Plate 6 Loop stoma with rod in position. Reproduced with permission

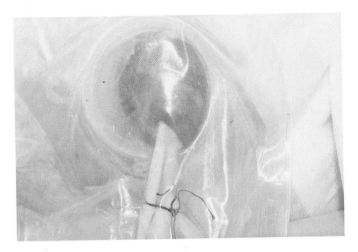

Plate 7 Urostomy with Ureteric stents. Reproduced with permission

of pouch aperture and educating the patient on skin care needs to be considered.

Contact dermatitis is an allergic or sensitive skin reaction to any part of the stoma bag. It is recognised by the symmetrical shape on the skin by the part of the bag affecting the skin. The treatment is to remove the irritant part which may necessitate a change in the appliance being used. If this is not acceptable barrier films, in spray, cream or wipe format, may be used to protect the skin. The use of hydrocolloid skin protective wafers provides an ideal environment to promote healing of sore or broken skin. In extreme cases a topical steroid may be required but this must be used with caution as the skin can become more fragile and more susceptible to skin problems in the future. Pre-operative patch testing of appliance adhesives may be indicated in patients known to have a sensitive skin (Burch 2004).

Prolapse of the stoma occurs when the bowel telescopes out of the skin opening making it longer in length. It is common in patients with a loop colostomy especially those with a transverse colostomy (Collett 2002). Either the distal or the proximal segment of the loop stoma can prolapse. The reason for this problem is due to inadequate fixing of the stoma to the abdominal wall at surgery (Lawson 2003). It is recommended that the stoma is sited through the rectus muscle to reduce the risk of stoma prolapse. Prolapse can be very distressing for the patient and they will need reassurance that the condition is not serious. They must also be aware that the swollen stoma is at risk of trauma and necrosis. The use of a larger appliance to incorporate the prolapse may be used. Placing baby oil inside the bag will help prevent friction between the stoma and bag. Surgery is not usually indicated unless the patient cannot tolerate it or if bowel obstruction or necrosis develops. Some prolapsed stomas can be reduced, this is achieved by applying a cold compress over the stoma or using an abdominal support belt without an opening (Borwell 1996).

Retraction of the stoma occurs when it recedes below the skin level owing to tension. It causes a 'moat' effect around the stoma and leakage problems can develop as a result. The cause of retraction can be weight gain, premature removal of the stoma rod or mucocutaneous separation (see also Table 5.1). This problem is effectively managed with the use of a convexity appliance or a seal to make the stoma protrude – this will achieve a secure seal around the stoma. A two-piece appliance with a belt will also help to ensure security.

Stenosis of the stoma occurs when the opening (lumen) narrows as a result of scar tissue forming from necrosis, infection, retraction or mucocutaneous separation. It can cause difficulty in passing stool and it pools around the stoma making the skin ulcerated and sore. In the long term surgical revision is necessary but the interim management is to advise colostomy patients to maintain a soft stool, using a stoma dilator regularly to dilate the opening or using a paste, seal or convexity appliance to maintain skin integrity (Collett 2002).

Granulomas have a 'cauliflower' appearance on the stoma. They are friable and bleed easily. These hyper-granulated lumps often develop where the sutures were inserted in the stoma and can appear many years after surgery. They mainly occur at the mucocutaneous junction or can appear on the surface of the stoma. Repeated trauma, such as friction from the stoma flange (base plate) can cause this problem. The treatment involves applying silver nitrate or surgical removal. Re-sizing the stoma bag aperture may be required to ensure there is no friction. Care must be taken to exclude cancerous growths or any other gastrointestinal disorder (Burch 2004).

Trauma to a stoma is rare, especially major trauma. It might result from a road traffic accident or self-mutilation of the stoma (Taylor 1995). Minor trauma can be caused by an ill-fitting appliance rubbing against the stoma, which in turn can cause mucosal ulceration. Applying a bag that fits correctly will allow the ulceration to heal. However, if the trauma has been caused by the patient's participation in contact sports or hobbies it is advisable they wear a stoma shield and belt for protection. Minor trauma to the parastomal skin can also occur due to folliculitis. This problem is more common in men and the regular removal of the parastomal hair by shaving should reduce this compliant (Collett 2002).

Pancaking occurs when there is no air in the bag resulting in negative pressure which makes its sides stick together. This prevents stool passing into the bag and causes it to collect at the top of the bag or around the stoma. This can result in the bag being 'pushed off' (Collett 2002). If the consistency of the stool is thick this can cause pancaking and dietary advice is needed. Patients are advised to place an adhesive patch over the bag filter to keep air within. Stoma accessories such as a stoma bridge or foam block can be used to prevent the sides of the bag sticking together. A small amount of baby oil or scrunched up tissue inside the bag can be effective (Burch 2004).

Odour and the fear of smelling unpleasant are of paramount importance and concern for the patient with a stoma. The only time odour should be detected is when the bag is emptied or changed. Various accessories such as deodorant sprays, drops or capsules can be placed in the bag to help eliminate odour. Air fresheners used before and after a bag change are helpful. Advising the patient to avoid certain foods can also help.

Table 7.1 identifies the variety of stoma care accessories that are available to help resolve the numerous physical problems related to stomas. It may be that one or a combination of these products is needed. It is important that a detailed assessment is performed to identify the problem to be able to initiate a change in stoma care management.

SUMMARY

Patients can experience a variety of physical problems with their stoma that can be distressing and embarrassing. Most of these problems can be treated by educating the patient and a change in the practical management of their stoma, although some will require surgery. The early recognition and treatment of these problems will ensure a better quality of life for the stoma patient.

Table 7.1 Stoma care accessories for physical problems related to stomas

Product	Problem/usage
Paste	Retracted stoma
	Crease/dips
Skin protective sprays, wipes or wafers	Effluent/contact dermatitis
Adhesive remover sprays or wipes	Residual adhesive from flange
Powder	Sore excoriated weeping skin
Deodorant sprays, drops or capsules	Eliminate odour
Abdominal support belt, corsets or girdles	Parastomal hernia
Convexity appliance	Retracted stoma
	Stenosis
Adhesive seals/washers	Retracted stoma
	Creases/dips
	Stenosis
Silver nitrate	Granulomas
Stoma dilator	Stenosis
Stoma shield	Prevent trauma to stoma
Stoma bridge/foam block	Pancaking

SELF-EVALUATION QUESTIONS AND ANSWERS

Questions

Mrs James is a 57-year-old lady who had a bowel operation two years ago resulting in the formation of an end colostomy. Over the past month she has noticed that her stoma is bleeding profusely while cleaning it as well as experiencing pain and discomfort. She has also noticed that there are lumps on her stoma.

1. What is causing the stoma to bleed?
2. What would you need to check/exclude before treatment commenced?
3. What is the treatment for this problem?
4. Why would you need to check that the appliance was fitting correctly?

Mr Arnold is a 62-year-old gentleman who has a transverse colostomy and is very anxious because he has noticed that his stoma has increased in size and length.

5. What is the problem with Mr Arnold's stoma?
6. What do you need to tell him?
7. What change would you make in his stoma management?
8. If surgery was needed what are the indications?

Answers

1. Granulomas

2. The lumps are not cancerous or any other gastrointestinal disease

3. Silver nitrate or surgery

4. An incorrect fitting appliance can rub against the stoma causing the granulomas

5. Prolapsed stoma

6. Reassure and explain to him that the condition is not serious or life threatening

7. Use a larger appliance to accommodate prolapse and add baby oil inside the bag to prevent friction

8. Surgery is required if the prolapse is causing necrosis or obstruction

REFERENCES

Black, P. (1997) Practical stoma care: a community approach. *British Journal of Community Health Nursing* **2**, 249–53.

Borwell, B. (1996) Managing stoma problems. Professional Nurse [wall chart], MacMillan Magazines Ltd, London.

Breeze, J. (2000) Stoma care – an update. *Pharmaceutical Journal* **265**, 823–6.

Burch, J. (2004) The management and care of people with stoma complications. *British Journal of Nursing* **13**, 307–18.

Collett, K. (2002) Practical aspects of stoma management. *Nursing Standard* **6**, 45–52.

Devlin, H. (1982) Stomatherapy review, part 3. *Coloproctology* **5**, 298–306.

Hughes, S & Irving, M. (1999) Intestinal stomas. In: D. Jones, ed. *ABC of Colorectal Diseases*, 2nd edn. BMJ Publishing Group, London.

Lawson, A. (2003) Complications of stomas. In: D.C. Elcoat, ed. *Stoma Care Nursing*. Hollister Ltd, Berkshire.

Lyon, C. & Smith, A. (2001) *Abdominal Stomas and Their Skin Disorders: An Atlas of Diagnosis and Management*. Martin Dunitz, London.

Myers, C. (1996) *Stoma Care Nursing: A Patient-Centred Approach*. Arnold, London.

Taylor, P. (1995) Stoma complications. In: P. Taylor, ed. *Stoma Care in the Community: A Clinical Resource for Practitioners*. NT Books, London.

Wade, B. (1989) *A Stoma is for Life*. Scutari Press, Harrow.

Changing a Stoma Appliance

8

Theresa Porrett

INTRODUCTION

Patients return to the ward from the operating theatre wearing a transparent drainable appliance, this type of appliance allows observation of the stoma (size and colour) and any output from the stoma to be observed and emptied. It can remain in place for four to five days postoperatively (Coloplast 1995). If the patient is mobile and able to go to the bathroom this is the best environment in which to change the appliance, it is private and once at home the patient will almost certainly change the appliance sitting or standing in the bathroom or sitting on the toilet (Porrett & Joels 1996). If the appliance change has to take place at the bedside ensure the patient's privacy with curtains well closed. If this is the first time the appliance will have been changed since surgery remember that the patient will have be nervous and will be closely observing you for your reaction to the stoma. Despite verbal reassurance, if your face shows disgust or anxiety, the patient will experience huge psychological damage (Dudas 1982, Ewing 1989).

The aim of this chapter is to understand the principles and practice of changing a stoma appliance.

LEARNING OBJECTIVES

By the end of the chapter the reader will be able to:

❏ list the items required to change an appliance;
❏ understand the differences in technique when changing a one- or two-piece appliance;

❏ cut an aperture in the flange to the correct size ensuring skin protection;

❏ describe how to empty a drainable appliance;

❏ understand the principles of correct disposal of used appliances.

TIMING OF APPLIANCE CHANGE

There is no set time when the appliance should be changed. At home patients tend to develop a routine particularly as they discover that there are periods when the stoma is less or more active. The urostomist will find that first thing in the morning, prior to drinking, is the most convenient time to change the appliance as less urine is produced. A colostomist will tend to change the appliance immediately or as soon as possible after the stoma has acted, which is often in the morning after they have eaten. An ileostomy tends to be at its least active about two hours after eating or first thing in the morning prior to breakfast and therefore this time will be more convenient as there is less chance of the stoma working while the appliance is being changed (Erwin-Toth & Doughty 1992).

If you have noted that an appliance is leaking it must be changed immediately to prevent skin excoriation and abdominal wound contamination. A nurse must never be tempted to try to seal the leaking appliance with extra tape or pads.

PROCEDURE FOR APPLIANCE CHANGE

Prior to starting to change the appliance, a number of preparations need to be made to ensure the procedure takes place in an organised and efficient manner:

• Assist the patient to sit or lie in a comfortable position or walk out to the bathroom if they are mobile.

• Ensure the patient's privacy is maintained at all times (Royal College of Nursing (RCN) 2002).

• Wash and dry your hands and put on an apron and gloves.

- Prepare warm water in the sink or in a bowl.
- Ensure you have:
  - soft cloths for cleaning and drying (not toilet paper) the new appliance;
  - scissors, if necessary, to cut flange opening to size;
  - disposable bag for used appliance and wipes;
  - deodorising spray – especially if changing appliance by the bedside;
  - any accessories the stoma care nurse (SCN) might have recommended (paste, washer, skin barrier cream) (Armstrong 2001, Trainor *et al.* 2003).

Procedure for changing a one-piece appliance (Elcoat 1986, Armstrong 2001, Trainor *et al.* 2003)

- Remove the used appliance, starting from the top of the adhesive and peeling downwards. Peel gently using two hands, one hand holding the appliance and the other supporting the skin to prevent trauma.
- Place the used appliance in a clinical waste bag (as per the hospital procedure for disposing of clinical waste). See Chapters 9 and 10 for disposal advice in the community.
- The skin surrounding the stoma should be gently cleansed using warm water and soft wipes (not toilet paper). Any faecal residue or mucus should be gently wiped from the stoma.
- The surrounding skin should be thoroughly dried using the soft wipes.
- The stoma should be measured and the appropriate size hole cut in the flange. The aperture should be 3mm larger than the stoma, no greater or skin will be exposed and become sore due to contact with the faeces or urine (Coloplast 1995).
- Remove the backing paper from the new appliance and place the opening in the flange over the stoma and firmly fix in place, ensuring there are no creases in the flange which could act as a gully allowing leakage.

- If a drainable appliance is being used the closure clip must be secured or the tap closed.

Procedure for changing a two-piece appliance (Armstrong 2001, Trainor *et al.* 2003)

- Remove the used appliance in one piece; do not detach the bag from the flange. Start from the top of the adhesive and peel downwards. Peel gently using two hands, one hand holding the appliance and the other supporting the skin to prevent trauma.
- Place the used appliance in a clinical waste bag (as per the hospital procedure for disposing of clinical waste).
- The skin surrounding the stoma should be gently cleansed using warm water and soft wipes (not toilet paper). Any faecal residue or mucus should be gently wiped from the stoma.
- The surrounding skin should be thoroughly dried using the soft wipes.
- The stoma should be measured and the appropriate size hole cut in the flange. The aperture should be 3 mm larger than the stoma, no greater or skin will be exposed and become sore due to contact from the faeces or urine.
- Remove the backing paper from the new flange and place the opening in the flange over the stoma and firmly fix in place, ensuring there are no creases in the flange which could act as a gully allowing leakage.
- Attach the appliance to the flange.
- If a drainable appliance is being used the closure clip must be secured or the tap closed.

Procedure for changing a one-piece appliance on a loop stoma that has a rod in place

- Remove the used appliance, starting from the top of the adhesive and peeling downwards. Peel gently using two

hands, one holding the appliance and the other supporting the skin to prevent trauma.

- Place the used appliance in a clinical waste bag (as per the hospital procedure for disposing of clinical waste).
- The skin surrounding the stoma should be gently cleansed using warm water and soft wipes (not toilet paper). Any faecal residue or mucus should be gently wiped from the stoma.
- The surrounding skin should be thoroughly dried using the soft wipes.
- The stoma should be measured and the appropriate size hole cut in the flange. The aperture should be 3 mm larger than the stoma, no greater or skin will be exposed and become sore due to contact from the faeces or urine. Never cut the hole in the flange large enough to expose the rod, as this will leave large areas of skin exposed and unprotected.
- Slide the rod so that the skin is exposed on one side of the stoma. Peel back the backing paper from one half of the flange and place this directly on the skin which has been exposed.
- Slide the rod in the opposite direction so that it now covers the positioned flange. Remove the backing paper and smooth the remaining flange onto the now exposed skin ensuring there are no creases in the flange which could act as a gully allowing leakage.
- Centralise the rod so that both ends are clearly visible and are sitting on top of the positioned flange.
- If a drainable appliance is being used the closure clip must be secured or the tap closed.

Once you have completed the practical aspects of the appliance change ensure that:

- the patient is offered a hand wash if they have participated in the procedure;
- a deodorising spray is used to leave no potentially embarrassing odours for the patient when the curtains are drawn;

- the patient is left comfortably positioned in bed if immobile or is escorted back to their bed area if mobile;
- you remove gloves and apron;
- you wash your hands;
- all supplies have been returned to the patient's locker;
- you document the procedure and report stoma appearance and skin condition.

Emptying an appliance at the bedside if the patient is immobile

- Place a protective pad under the drainable end of the appliance and position the clip over the jug.
- Remove clip and empty contents into jug.
- Clean the end of the appliance using dry toilet paper or tissue.
- Securely replace the clip.
- Remove protective pad.
- Use deodorising spray to remove residual odour.
- Dispose stomal output down the sluice.
- Document stomal output on fluid balance chart.
- Remove gloves and apron and wash hands.

Although it is acknowledged that the SCN is primarily responsible for teaching the patient self-care in preparation for discharge home (RCN 2002), there will be occasions when the ward nurse is required to assist the patient in an appliance change as part of the patient's self-care learning. It is possible to use Orem's nursing model and apply this to aiding self-care with particular reference to stoma care (Ewing 1989, Table 8.1).

Table 8.1 Orem's nursing model as applied to stoma care patient teaching (Ewing 1989)

Orems's helping methods (1980)	Examples applied to stoma care teaching
Acting for another	Changing the appliance for the patient because they are unable to undertake this hygiene/elimination need for themselves
Teaching	Showing the patient how each part of the procedure should be done and explaining why, e.g. showing the patient how to dry the peri-stomal skin thoroughly to ensure good adhesion of the flange
Guiding	The nurse prompts the patient to undertake a part/all of the procedure themselves, e.g. instructing the patient on how to support the skin when removing an appliance
Supporting	The nurse being present in the bathroom while the patient undertakes the appliance change themselves with the nurse providing psychological support only
Providing a developmental environment	Ensuring the appliance change or appliance emptying takes place in a private/safe environment with maintenance of the patient's dignity Ensuring the nurse does not display any disgust at odour or stomal appearance

SELF-EVALUATION QUESTIONS AND ANSWERS

Questions

1. What items are required to change an appliance?

2. When might the best time be to change an appliance for a urostomist?

3. Following an appliance change at the patient's bedside what is the role of the nurse post procedure?

4. How do you correctly cut a flange to size?

5. How do you correctly dispose of a used stoma appliance in hospital, and is this procedure different from at home?

Answers

1. Warm water in the sink or a bowl, soft cloths, new appliance, scissors, disposable bag, deodorising spray, gloves and any accessories the SCN might have recommended.

2. The urostomist will find that first thing in the morning prior to drinking is the most convenient time to change the appliance as less urine is produced.

3. The role of the nurse is to ensure that the patient is comfortable, no odour is left remaining, all clinical waste is correctly disposed of, supplies are returned to the patient's locker and the procedure is documented (stomal appearance, skin condition, amount of stomal output).

4. The flange should be cut so that the aperture is no more than 3 mm larger than the stoma; this ensures the peri-stomal skin is protected. All appliances come with a cutting guide to help you measure the size and shape of the stoma and often the SCN will have left a template of the stoma size for you to use.

5. In hospital all clinical waste is disposed of in a clinical waste bag. At home the patient is advised to empty the appliance, seal in a disposable plastic bag and place in the bin.

REFERENCES

Armstrong, E. (2001) Practical aspects of stoma care. *Nursing Times* **97**, 40–2.

Coloplast Ltd. (1995) *Ostomy and Ostomy Patients*. Coloplast Ltd, Peterborough.

Dudas, S. (1982) Postoperative considerations. In: D.C. Broadwell & B.S. Jackson, eds. *Principles of Ostomy Care*. CV Mosby, St Louis.

Elcoat, C. (1986) *Stoma Care Nursing*, p. 86–7. Ballière Tindall, London.

Ewing, G. (1989) The nursing preparation of stoma patients for self care. *Journal of Advanced Nursing* **14**, 411–20.

Erwin-Toth, P. & Doughty, D. (1992) Principles and procedures of stomal management. In: B. Hampton & R. Bryant, eds. *Ostomies and Continent Diversions*. Mosby Year Book, St Louis.

Porrett, T. & Joels, J. (1996) Continuing care in the community. In: C. Myers, ed. *Stoma Care Nursing: A Patient Centred Approach.* Arnold, London.

Royal College of Nursing (2002) *RCN Standards of Care – Colorectal and Stoma Care Nursing.* RCN, London.

Trainor, B., Thompson, M., Boyd-Carson, W. & Boyd, K. (2003) Changing an appliance. *Nursing Standard* **18**, 41–2.

9 Discharge Planning and Supporting Patient Self-Care

Antoinette Johnson & Theresa Porrett

INTRODUCTION

Discharge planning and teaching patients to care for their stoma themselves is an integral part of rehabilitating the stoma patient. Discharge planning should begin at the time the patient is admitted to hospital and the practical teaching of the patient to be self-caring for their stoma will start in the post-operative period.

For patients entering hospital to have stoma forming surgery, the need for physical, psychological and social adjustment will continue when they are discharged into the community. Therefore, a comprehensive and individualised discharge plan is essential to ensure that all their practical and emotional needs are met (Curry, 1991).

With the ever-increasing trend today for a shorter stay in hospital due to advances in surgical techniques and political and managerial agendas, teaching patients to be self-caring with their stoma is a key element in their discharge planning.

The aim of this chapter is for the reader to understand the principles and practice of an effective discharge plan and teaching patients to be self-caring for their stoma.

LEARNING OBJECTIVES

By the end of this chapter the reader will be able to:

❏ discuss the integral part that discharge planning plays in the rehabilitation of the stoma patient;
❏ understand the importance of practical teaching for the stoma patient to achieve self care;

❏ discuss the measures needed to prepare a stoma patient for discharge;

❏ recognise that continuity of care should be seamless from hospital to community setting.

ROLE OF THE STOMA CARE NURSE (SCN) IN DISCHARGE PLANNING AND REHABILITATING THE STOMA PATIENT

When patients are discharged from the safe and secure environment of the hospital they have to deal with adapting back into the community, resuming daily activities and re-integrating into social groups.

Even with good pre operative counselling and effective practical teaching of basic stoma care, many patients do not fully realise the true impact of stoma surgery until they have been discharged from hospital.

(Brady 1980)

Therefore, the role of the SCN is to ensure that patients are prepared for discharge and are rehabilitated back into the community. This liaison and co-ordination role is key to the continuing care of the stoma patient from hospital to home. The role of the SCN in discharge planning and rehabilitating the stoma patient is varied and includes:

• providing holistic individualised care;
• planning patient care which is focused on the achievement of self-care;
• direct delivery of care, providing information and teaching new skills;
• an in-depth knowledge of the physical, psychological and emotional effects of stoma formation surgery;
• co-ordination of care within the multidisciplinary team;
• providing continuity of care following discharge with telephone contact and home visits;
• measuring and evaluating the outcomes of interventions.

SUPPORTING PATIENT SELF-CARE

Teaching practical stoma management is essential to facilitate the patient's discharge back into the community. Teaching the patient practical skills in caring for their stoma improves their independence; this emphasis on gaining practical skills reflects patients' wishes for learning (Kelly & Henry 1992). Co-ordinated care and effective communication are crucial because of the short stay in hospital following surgery and the need to teach the patient the practical skills of stoma management prior to discharge.

Ewing's (1989) study investigated the nursing preparation of stoma patients for self care and identified nine tasks associated with the physical care of the stoma (Table 9.1). The study also found that many patients did not progress to 'unsupervised completion of the whole procedure'. Part of the problem was attributed to unco-ordinated care. Patients would be allowed to participate dependant upon the nursing involvement. To resolve the variable involvement of the patients, Ewing suggested the use of a check-list in conjunction with the nursing care plans to provide a more co-ordinated and progressive teaching approach (see Fig. 9.1).

Table 9.1 Practical aspects of stoma care

Nine aspects of the physical care of the stoma
Preparation of the equipment
Preparation of the patient
Removal of the old appliance
Skin care
Skin protection
Selection of a new appliance
Preparation of the new appliance
Application
Disposal

Name...

Stoma type...

Date of surgery..

Name and size of appliance..

Frequency of bag change...

Please tick and date
1. Able to fasten clip on bag
2. Can empty bag with supervision and fasten clip
3. Has observed stoma
4. Can identify all equipment needed to take to bathroom for bag change
5. Prepares the new bag
6. Removes the soiled bag
7. Cleans and dries skin around stoma
8. Reapply new bag   Accessories...   ....
9. Disposal of soiled bag and wipes
10. Whole procedure under supervision
11. Whole procedure without supervision
Any problems please contact the Stoma Care Nurse on

Fig. 9.1 Discharge planning check-list for self-care of stoma

Before teaching commences, it is important to consider patients' mental and physical abilities and accept that there will be some who will never be able to achieve self-care. It is also essential to provide a conducive learning environment by providing privacy and minimising distractions and interruptions.

Prior to discharge the patient should be able to complete all the tasks in the check-list, i.e. be able to change the appliance correctly unaided.

Patients may also find it useful to have written instructions to help them learn the stages involved in changing their appliance. These instructions should be clear and concise, and can enhance practical teaching but are not an alternative to the hands-on practice that patients need (Davenport 2003). Figure 9.2 gives an example of written instructions.

Things to get ready
- A new stoma bag cut to size
- Bowl or sink of water
- Wipes
- Disposable bag
- Air freshener

What to do
- Have all the above items ready
- Cut your new bag to size if it has not already been done
- Remove the old bag, fold it in half to seal the contents and place in the disposable bag
- Clean firmly but gently the skin around the stoma with wipes moistened in warm water
- Dry skin thoroughly
- At this stage you might want to cover the stoma with a wipe in case it should work
- Apply new bag, remembering to remove backing
- Check it is sealed completely
- Place disposable bag in the bin

Fig. 9.2 Patient check-sheet for use at home

DISCHARGE PLANNING GOALS

Learning the practical management of stoma care is not the only issue for patients prior to discharge. The patient needs to be informed and confident about many other aspects of stoma care such as:

- when to empty or change the appliance;
- how to open and close the appliance if using a drainable appliance;
- how to look after the skin around the stoma;
- knowledge of how to correctly dispose of equipment in the community.

It is the role of the SCN, in conjunction with ward staff, to ensure that the patient is fully informed of the discharge advice. This advice will need to be continued and/or reinforced in the community setting. Patients need to be aware of possible complications that may occur with the stoma. These include:

- skin excoriation;
- slight bleeding from stoma;
- shrinkage in the size of the stoma;
- leakages;
- diarrhoea and constipation;
- retraction of stoma;
- prolapse;
- herniation;
- stenosis.

When the patient has been taught to recognise and understand these problems and knows they have to contact the SCN promptly for further advice, the foundations of skills and knowledge needed prior to going home will have been built. Preparation for leaving hospital can be a stressful time for patients, often the key concern is how they will obtain supplies once they leave hospital. Therefore, the SCN will ensure that patients leave hospital knowing how to:

- correctly store their appliances;
- contact the SCN;
- contact the district nurse;
- obtain stoma supplies in the community.

Prior to discharge patients have many concerns about how the stoma will affect their daily life and advice and information from the SCN will focus on the following areas:

- diet;
- hygiene;
- clothing;
- returning to work;
- recreational activities/hobbies;
- changes in their physical relationship;
- travelling considerations/constraints;
- local and national support groups
  - British Colostomy Association;
  - Ileostomy Association;
  - Urostomy Association.

More information regarding these issues can be found in Chapter 10 and the Appendix on page 169.

COMMUNITY FOLLOW-UP

The transition from hospital to home can be a stressful period for the stoma patient. The importance of community care is well documented but this transition has been seen as a weak link in the care of a stoma patient (Allison 1996). This is attributed to fragmented visits and poor communication (Black 2000).

Following discharge from the hospital the SCN will visit the patient at home to maintain continuity of care. It is also important to inform the patient's general practitioner (GP), district nurse and other community services of any relevant information to ensure a cohesive approach to the patient's care at home (Taylor 2003). The SCN should ideally visit the patient within

48 hours following discharge but it can be up to a week. On visiting the patient at home the SCN assesses how well the patient is adapting to life with a stoma by observing the following:

- the general condition of the patient's home;
- the patient's ability to change the appliance at home;
- the patient's feelings/emotions;
- the patient's appearance and cleanliness;
- the patient's eating and elimination habits;
- the patient's interaction with family/friends;
- resumed work/recreational/social/sporting activities;
- re-established physical relationship.

Assessing the patient on these visits will give the SCN a view on how well the patient is adapting at home and highlight any potential problems that can be acted upon promptly. Depending upon the problem it may be appropriate to seek advice from other allied healthcare professionals, e.g. social worker, occupational therapist, GP.

How well the patient is adapting at home will influence the frequency of home visits required. Home visits can be curtailed once the patient has adjusted sufficiently and regained their independence. However, it can take up to a year or more before the patient has fully adjusted to life with a stoma. It is important that the patients know that even when formal home visits have been stopped they can contact the SCN at any time for advice and support. Other opportunities when the SCN can monitor patients' rehabilitation progress include seeing them at their follow-up clinic appointments, at support group meetings or by carrying out regular phone checks.

SELF-EVALUATION QUESTIONS AND ANSWERS

Questions

1. Describe, in order, the practical steps required for the patient to be self-sufficient with stoma care.

2. When should discharge planning commence?

3. What advice should the patient be given prior to discharge on potential stoma complications?

4. When should practical stoma teaching start and what is the benefit to the patient?

5. What is the role of the SCN in discharge planning?

Answers

1. The patient should demonstrate that they can identify when the bag needs to be emptied or changed; can empty the bag if it is a drainable bag; can change the bag independently; can demonstrate good skin care practices; and show correct disposal of equipment.

2. Discharge planning should start when the patient is admitted to hospital as this allows for problems to be identified and a care plan implemented to resolve them.

3. Stoma complications can be divided into short- and long-term problems. Short-term problems include skin excoriation, slight bleeding from stoma, shrinkage in the size of the stoma, leakages and diarrhoea/constipation. Long-term problems include retraction of stoma, prolapse, herniation and stenosis.

4. Teaching a patient to care for their stoma should start in the postoperative period. This will promote confidence and independence in the patient enabling them to return home.

5. The role of the SCN is to co-ordinate an individualised holistic care plan for stoma patients within the multidisciplinary team and ensuring that this care is continued in the community setting.

REFERENCES

Allison, M. (1996) Discharge planning for the person with a stoma. In: C. Myers, ed. *Stoma Care Nursing*. Arnold, London.

Black, P. (2000) *Holistic Stoma Care*. Baillière Tindall, London.

Brady, V.A. (1980) Community care of the stoma patients. *Nursing* **1**, 741.

Curry, A. (1991) Returning home with confidence. Discharge planning in stoma care: a conceptual framework. *Professional Nurse* **6**, 536–9.

Davenport, R. (2003) Post operative stoma care. In: D.C. Elcoat, ed. *Stoma Care Nursing*. Hollister Ltd, Berkshire.

Ewing, G. (1989) The nursing preparation of stoma patients for self care. *Journal of Advanced Nursing* **14**, 411–20.

Kelly, M. & Henry, T. (1992) A thirst for practical knowledge: stoma patients' opinions of the service they receive. *Professional Nurse* **7**, 350–6.

Taylor, P. (2003) Community aspects of stoma care. In: D.C. Elcoat, ed. *Stoma Care Nursing*. Hollister Ltd, Berkshire.

10 Questions Commonly Asked by the Patient with a Newly Formed Stoma

Theresa Porrett

INTRODUCTION

Following stoma forming surgery patients will have many questions about the stoma and how it might affect their lifestyle, work and social activities. Some of the questions commonly asked by patients are discussed in this chapter. The advice outlined in the answers is general in nature and if you have any doubts or concerns about an individual patient's queries it is essential that you involve the stoma care nurse (SCN). Equally, if patients have specific concerns regarding their stoma management or surgery you should advise the patient to discuss these with their SCN or the consultant who performed their surgery as they will be able to advise the patient more specifically, bearing in mind the underlying condition and the surgical procedure performed.

LEARNING OBJECTIVES

By the end of this chapter the reader will be able to:

❏ discuss the main issues and concerns experienced by patients following stoma formation;
❏ explain the national and local support mechanisms available to stoma patients;
❏ identify the clinical staff who can support patients and address any specific concerns they may raise.

COMMONLY ASKED QUESTIONS

Patients have many information needs and will be given a large amount of information at all stages of their treatment

(Royal College of Nursing (RCN) 2002). This information will be both written and verbal but will require reinforcement and clarification (Mead 1994; Black 1997a). Written information is essential to consolidate what patients have been told. The majority of appliance manufacturers and national ostomy support groups produce booklets summarising the basics of stoma surgery and stoma management.

Will I have to alter my diet or avoid certain foods?

Following stoma surgery patients often think they will have to totally change their diet and severely restrict their food intake. This is not the case but patients need to be aware of minor alterations that they may need to make to their food and fluid input following surgery. When discussing food with patients try to avoid using the term 'diet' as this can be interpreted negatively by many patients as meaning rigid restrictions to their diet or that they have to be on a 'special diet' now that they have a stoma.

The main concern for ostomists is that certain foods can cause a change in stool consistency or an increase in wind and odour. It is essential that ostomists experiment with their food intake and do not exclude an item from their diet after having tried it once only. Initially after surgery many foods may cause increased wind but after a few months many ostomists find they can eat what they perceived initially to be problematic foods with no problems. Therefore, the key to a healthy diet for the ostomist is experimentation with food. Rigid instructions are impossible to give as everybody reacts differently to and likes different foods (Farbrother 1993). There are NO foods which MUST be avoided or excluded from the ostomist's diet.

General dietary tips for the ostomist (Bradley 1997):

- Chew food thoroughly.
- Try to eat three meals a day at regular times.
- Drink a minimum of eight cups of fluid per day.
- Ensure fruit and vegetables are included in the diet.

- When trying new foods for the first time after surgery try a small portion first and then gradually increase to a normal size serving.
- If on first eating a food causes wind, do not exclude it from your diet, wait a few weeks and then try again.

Foods which can cause excess wind formation in the ostomist with a faecal stoma include:

- beer;
- brussel sprouts;
- cabbage;
- cauliflower;
- cucumber;
- eggs;
- beans;
- onions;
- spicy foods.

The following can help reduce wind production:

- Do not talk while eating.
- Avoid drinking through a straw.
- Avoid fizzy drinks (pour drinks into a glass to get rid of some of the bubbles and let it stand for five minutes or so before drinking).
- Eat regularly and do not miss meals.
- Eat slowly.
- Natural yoghurt.
- Peppermint tea (Collett 2002).

For a colostomist there really are no dietary restrictions but the ileostomist should be aware of a number of issues:

- An ileostomist will lose more water and salt through their ileostomy output than prior to their surgery (as they no longer reabsorb water from the colon) and therefore they will need to drink around eight to ten cups of fluid per day to make up for this loss, equally they will need to add extra salt to their food on the plate and use salt in cooking (Black 1997b).

- Certain foods, which are very high in fibre and poorly digested, can temporarily 'block' the stoma. Therefore, all high fibre foods such as nuts, celery, and sweetcorn should be chewed well (Farbrother 1993).

For the urostomist there is no special dietary advice but there are some guidelines regarding their fluid and food intake:

- Fish and asparagus can give the urine an unusual odour.
- A glass of cranberry juice a day can reduce the amount of mucus produced by the stoma.
- Foods high in vitamin C (such as oranges) can help keep the urine more acid which can help prevent urinary tract infections.
- If the urine appears dark it is a sign that the urine is becoming concentrated and the urostomist needs to drink more fluid to ensure the urine remains dilute.

Can I drink alcohol now that I have a stoma?
Alcohol can be included as part of a healthy diet for all ostomists. Gassy drinks such as beer can cause wind. It is advisable to adhere to the recommended alcohol intake of two to three units per day for women and three to four units per day for men. Regular consumption above this recommended level becomes detrimental to health. One unit of alcohol is equal to one pub measure of spirit or half a pint of beer/lager. It is not advisable to save up units to have 'a big night out'. If the ostomist does overindulge they may have problems with emptying or changing the appliance, which could cause leakage or spillage problems.

Can I play sports?
Generally patients should be advised to avoid strenuous exercise and lifting for six weeks after their operation to allow the wound to fully heal, but during this time walking is a good

and safe form of exercise. There is a risk of incisional hernia formation following any abdominal surgery and therefore it is important that patients do not commence strenuous exercise or lifting prior to this to ensure that the abdominal muscles have fully healed (Coloplast 1995). Once the patient has been reviewed by their surgeon in the outpatient department, usually six to eight weeks after their operation, they will be given the all clear to start exercising fully again. Participation in contact sports is possible with a stoma but it is important to avoid any direct trauma to the stoma. A plastic stomal cap is available, which protects the stoma from trauma. This is placed over the stoma, on top of the appliance and is held in place by an elasticated belt. The SCN can arrange a stomal cap for patients and will advise on its use. Swimming is a good exercise, it is advisable for patients to eat lightly prior to swimming and ensure the pouch is emptied just before swimming. There are a variety of small pouches, which are ideal for sporting activities, and the SCN can supply samples of these for patients to try. There is also a range of swimwear with internal pockets to both support and disguise the appliance. A number of companies manufacture these, and again the SCN can provide the appropriate details. For those who engage in vigorous exercise there are additional belts, which may be worn to support the stoma and the appliance. If the patient has any doubts at all they should discuss their concerns with the SCN prior to commencing any new sporting activities.

Can I wear my normal clothes?

It is advisable for patients to wear snug fitting underclothes. If the appliance is placed inside the pants it supports the pouch and prevents movement of the appliance when the patient moves. Modification to clothing should be minimal if at all. It is important that belts or very firm waistbands do not cross directly over the stoma as this may cause trauma to the stoma. If the waistband lies directly over the stoma men may be advised to wear braces and not a belt. Some patients will slightly alter their style of dress, e.g. by wearing skirts or trousers with front pleats to disguise the stoma. It is fine for women to wear tights and if they wish to wear a tight fitting panty girdle these can be made specifically for them with an aperture for the appliance so that the faecal / urinary output can flow into the appliance freely. These girdles can be arranged through the SCN. The patient will quite naturally need time to rebuild confidence in their body image and at first may restrict themselves to baggy clothing. Initially this may be more comfortable because of the abdominal wound but patients should be encouraged to try their normal clothing. Should it be necessary, several manufacturers have designed items of clothing specifically for the ostomist, e.g. high-waisted trousers. The SCN will be able to give the patient specific information about these items. Once wearing their normal clothing, patients quickly realise that the appliance is not noticeable and this will of course help boost their confidence and self esteem.

Can I go back to work?

The majority of patients can return to their work environment. After stoma forming surgery it is reasonable to assume that as long as the patient is not undergoing any further treatment (such as chemotherapy) they should be able to return to work in approximately 12–16 weeks. Patients should be advised to keep an 'emergency' supply of all items required for a bag change at work. Often patients are worried about changing or emptying their appliance in a public toilet. Many patients are worried about leaving 'tell-tale' odours in the toilet and the SCN can provide the patient with a deodoriser to ensure this concern is minimised. If the patient's occupation involves rigorous activity or heavy lifting the patient should consult their doctor prior to returning to work (Coloplast 1995).

Can I take my pouch off in the bath or shower?

It is safe for patients to remove their appliance before bathing and showering. Often patients are concerned that bath water will enter the stoma but this is not the case. It is a matter of personal choice for patients but if they choose to keep the appliance on during bathing the appliance will need to be patted dry with a towel afterwards. Appliances are waterproof and the security of the adhesive is not reduced if it gets wet.

Where do I get my supplies?

While in hospital all the patient's stoma supplies will be provided by the SCN. Appliances are free to all patients over the age of 60 but younger patients will require an exemption certificate (P11). The SCN will arrange for the patient to obtain a prescription exemption application form and this will require signing by the patient's GP. At home patients have a choice of how they order their supplies once they have a prescription. They can take the prescription to a chemist; supplies will not be in stock but will be obtained by the chemist within a couple of days. Alternatively, they may use a home delivery service. The prescription details are placed in a pre-paid envelope and posted off to the delivery company, the supplies are then delivered to the patient's door. For older patients this service has many advantages as they do not have to walk to the chemist or carry bulky supplies home, equally many home delivery companies will arrange repeat prescriptions directly with the patient's GP. If the patient feels they would like to use a home delivery service the SCN can arrange this (Mead 1994).

How do I dispose of my used stoma appliance?

The recommended method of disposal is to empty the contents of the appliance down the toilet, seal the used appliance in a plastic bag and place it in the household bin (Mead 1994).

Can I go away on holiday?

Patients often worry about managing their stoma away from their home environment and will need encouragement and reassurance. Often just talking through their concerns will be enough to reassure them. There is no reason why a person with a stoma may not travel abroad or take a holiday. There are travel certificates available in many languages explaining that the patient has a medical condition and is carrying medical supplies in their hand luggage. This is particularly useful at Customs and avoids embarrassing bag searches. This certificate is available from the SCN. Patients should be advised to take double the amount of equipment that they would normally use for that period of time (to allow for any emergencies or increased appliance changes caused by travellers' diarrhoea) and to ensure it is carried in their hand luggage (Coloplast 1995). This avoids any worries about luggage not arriving with the patient at their destination. The only potential problem with flying is that everybody tends to produce more wind due to the changes in cabin pressure. Avoiding fizzy drinks while on the journey can help minimise wind production and the use of an appliance with a flatus filter can avoid the appliance filling with wind. It might be advisable to book an aisle seat to allow easy access to the toilets during the flight. As with any travellers there is a risk of 'travellers' diarrhoea' caused by the change in climate, food and water in a foreign country. Patients should be advised to drink bottled water and to increase their water and salt consumption in hot weather. Avoid ice cubes and salads, which may have been washed in tap water. Highly spiced foods should be treated with some caution especially if the patient is not used to eating them at home.

If diarrhoea is a problem while on holiday the advice to an ostomist would be very similar to the general advice anyone would receive:

- Drink plenty of water to replace what's being lost.
- Replace the salt and potassium lost by adding salt to food and drink fruit juices and savoury drinks. Over-the-counter oral re-hydration products can be used.
- Use an anti-diarrhoeal drug which can now be bought over the counter at chemist shops.

With regard to travel insurance it is essential that patients check with their insurer to ensure that pre-existing medical conditions are not excluded from the insurance. The relevant ostomy support group will be able to advise on suitable travel insurance companies.

When can I drive again?

Patients can usually resume driving six to eight weeks after surgery. Normally the surgeon will say that once a patient feels they are able to do an emergency stop it is safe for them to drive. It usually takes about six weeks for the patient to feel comfortable to do this and you can suggest that once a patient can stamp their foot with no abdominal pain they can drive. Patients may be concerned about the seat belt rubbing on the stoma. Products are available that hold the seat belt away from the abdomen (therefore stopping any friction/rubbing on the stoma). These can be bought from car accessory shops.

Are there any support groups available for people with a stoma?

In the UK there are a number of both national and local support groups and charities (see Appendix). The SCN will ensure that the patient is fully aware of the groups which are appropriate to them. Membership of these organisations can provide many benefits for patients, not least of these are social interaction and peer support. These organisations also produce very informative newsletters and information sheets, members are sent these periodically and they help to keep patients up to date especially regarding the availability and development of new stoma products.

Who should I tell about my stoma?

One of the main concerns for the ostomist is the issue of 'Who to tell' and 'How to tell' about their stoma. Initially patients may only wish their partner/close family members to know. As a person becomes more confident in the management of their stoma and begins to resume their usual social and work activities they may wish to tell others about their stoma. There is no right or wrong way to do this and often patients find it useful to role-play the discussion they wish to have. This is something that the SCN will be able to facilitate and support (Coloplast 1995). The key to remember is that if something is presented positively and without embarrassment that is how it will be perceived by the person receiving the news.

The young person without an established sexual relationship will need advice on how and when to tell their new 'partner' about the stoma. If social interaction is severely curtailed because of 'fear' of the stoma referral to other sources of advice, such as psychosexual counsellors, may be beneficial.

Can I still have sexual intercourse?

Naturally many ostomists are anxious about resuming sexual activity. Much of this anxiety stems from concerns about their change in body image and attractiveness to their partner. Reassurance should be given that sexual activity will not hurt the stoma. Practical suggestions can be given to the patient to reduce anxiety, such as:

- Empty the appliance prior to sexual activity.
- Use of a small appliance, stomal cap or appliance cover can lessen the presence of the appliance.
- The appliance may be rolled up to make it smaller and taped down so that it does not move.

Men may have concerns about or problems with impotence due to damage to the nerves during pelvic surgery (Bradley 1997). This can be discussed with the surgeon; many options are now available to treat this problem. Women may experience discomfort on deep penenetration and the SCN will be able to discuss with them changes in sexual positions or the use of extra vaginal lubricants (Bryant 1993).

Initially concerns about sexual activity centre around issues regarding the change in body image following surgery.

Following major abdominal surgery it is likely that many patients will experience a decrease in libido. As their general health improves, for many so does their libido, and it is at this stage that the SCN will be able to answer questions they might have and support the patient and their partner to be open in discussing their concerns and feelings. Patients often find it easier to discuss these intimate concerns with the SCN with whom they have developed a trusting relationship and therefore any concerns or issues raised by the patient are often best referred to the SCN. If sexual problems persist, there are a number of external support agencies such as Relate, SPOD (Sexual problems of the disabled) and the British Association of Sexual and Marital Therapy (see Appendix) that may be able to help.

Can I become pregnant now I've had a stoma?

Women with a stoma can become pregnant and have a normal pregnancy. Patients requiring contraception or wishing to discuss conception would be best advised to see their consultant or GP. Patients with an ileostomy may not be able to use the oral contraceptive pill as it may be excreted without being fully absorbed. Any surgery to the pelvic floor can alter the anatomy, which may make the use of the intra-uterine device (IUD) or cap difficult.

Some women who have had severe pelvic sepsis (Crohn's disease) may experience fertility problems but for the majority of women with a stoma fertility is unaffected. Some women may be advised by their obstetrician to have a caesarian section.

What can I do to prevent odour?

Without doubt this is the most common worry of patients with a stoma (Taylor 1995). Modern appliances are made of layers of bonded plastic and are odour proof. If the flange becomes displaced or the seal is detached, odour will escape from the bag. During an appliance change or emptying of the appliance there will be odour but patients need to be reassured that this is taking place in the toilet or bathroom, where people usually open their bowels and there is odour (Collett 2002). Domestic air fresheners mask odour and are commonly used in toilets/bathrooms. There are also deodoriser sprays available, which leave no odour. Patients have reported that striking a match in the toilet dispels odour. The matchstick can then be flushed down the toilet leaving no evidence. Alongside the deodoriser sprays the SCN can suggest and are available on prescription are a number of drops/pellets which can be placed in the appliance prior to use and help deodorise once emptied.

Flatus filters allow air to come out of the appliance so that it does not distend and become visible. These are made of charcoal to deodorise the flatus as it leaves the appliance so no tell-tale odour is noticeable (Black 1997b).

Now that I have a stoma will anything come out of my back passage?

The answer to this question will depend entirely on the type of surgery the patient has had. If they have had an abdominoperineal excision of rectum and formation of colostomy or a panproctocolectomy their rectum and anus has been surgically removed and therefore there is no remaining orifice.

If patients still have part of their rectum or anus they will continue to pass mucus (the bowel's natural lubricant). They can often have the sensation of wanting to have their bowels open and should be advised to sit on the toilet and push gently to expel any mucus. If they do this once or twice a day it will prevent a build up of mucus and therefore prevent the sensation of wanting to have their bowels open.

If the patient has a loop (or double-barrel stoma) it is possible for some faecal matter to by-pass the appliance and pass into the defunctioned loop of bowel. This occurs rarely but may result in the patient passing small amounts of stool per rectum.

Will any medicines I take affect the way my stoma works?

Many drugs can affect stomal function and some medications will not be completely absorbed (Davy & Porrett 2001). (Table 10.1 outlines the pharmacological considerations for stoma patients.) Patients should be advised to discuss this issue with their SCN or GP prior to commencing any new medications.

Table 10.1 Pharmacological considerations for stoma patients (Watkins 1987; Black 2000)

Drug	Possible effect on stoma
Antibiotics	May cause diarrhoea as they interfere with normal gut flora and cause the effluent to be green in colour
Anti-depressants/ anti-psychotics	May cause constipation in the colostomist. Laxatives and/or stool softeners may be used in conjunction with these drugs
Analgesics containing codeine/opiates	May cause constipation and often laxatives and/or stool softeners may be used in conjunction in the colostomist
Any enteric-coated or sustained-release drug	Probably ineffective, particularly in the ileostomist as not fully absorbed
Iron	Will darken the colour of the stool to black
Antacids	May make colostomy and ileostomy output grey in colour
Amitriptyline	Can cause urine to have a blue-green colour
Metronidazole	Can turn urine a reddish-brown colour
Senna	Can turn urine yellow/brown
Warfarin	Can turn urine orange

SELF-EVALUATION QUESTIONS AND ANSWERS

Questions

1. Why might an ileostomy stop functioning?
   A. Excessive fluid intake
   B. Allergy
   C. Mucocutaneous separation
   D. Food blockage

2. Mr Smith is a 50-year-old gentleman with an ileostomy. His wife is concerned that he will need a special liquid diet. What do you advise her?
   A. To restrict diet to fish and mashed potatoes
   B. To stop eating all fruit
   C. To eat a natural, well-balanced diet
   D. To puree all vegetables

3. Which of the following agencies would you not advise Mr Smith to contact regarding further information, advice and help with his stoma?
   A. Stoma care nurse specialist
   B. Local stoma support group
   C. Ileostomy and internal pouch support group
   D. The Urostomy Association

4. Which foods are thought to cause excess wind formation in the ostomist with a faecal stoma?

5. A colostomist asks you about ways in which they might reduce flatus production. What could you suggest to them?

6. What type of foods may block an ileostomy?

7. A 25-year-old man with a colostomy asks you if he can return to swimming now he has a stoma. What would you advise him?

8. How can a patient obtain their stoma supplies once they have a prescription?

9. An ostomist asks you if it is okay to put his appliance supplies in his suitcase when he is travelling abroad by plane. How do you advise him?

10. A long-standing urostomist calls you to inform you that they are being started on amitriptyline and are concerned it might affect the stoma. What would you advise the patient regarding the use of this medication?

Answers

1. D
2. C
3. D

4. Beer, brussel sprouts, cabbage, cauliflower, cucumber, eggs, beans, onions, spicy foods

5. The following can help reduce wind production:
   - Do not talk while eating
   - Avoid drinking through a straw
   - Avoid fizzy drinks
   - Eat regularly and do not miss meals
   - Eat slowly
   - Natural yoghurt and peppermint tea

6. Foods which are very high in fibre and poorly digested can temporarily 'block' the stoma. Therefore, high-fibre foods such as nuts, celery, and sweetcorn should be chewed well.

7. Swimming is a good exercise, it is advisable for patients to eat lightly prior to swimming and ensure the pouch is emptied just before swimming. There are a variety of small pouches, which are ideal for sporting activities, and the SCN can supply samples of these for patients to try. There is also a range of swimwear with internal pockets to both support and disguise the appliance. Many companies manufacture these, and the SCN can provide the appropriate details.

8. Once the patient has a prescription from the GP there are two methods of obtaining the appliances. The first is to take the prescription to the chemist as normal – they will not have the products in stock but will order them for collection by the patient one or two days later. The alternative is to use a home delivery service. The prescription is placed in a pre-paid envelope and supplies

are delivered to the patient's door. The SCN can arrange this service if the patient prefers this method.

9. Patients should be advised to take double the amount of equipment that they would normally use for that period of time (to allow for any emergencies or increased appliance changes caused by travellers' diarrhoea) and to ensure it is carried in their hand luggage. This avoids any worries about luggage not arriving with the patient at their destination.

10. Amitriptyline may cause the urine to have a blue/green colour but it is safe to take with a urostomy.

REFERENCES

Black, P. (1997a) Life carries on: stoma aftercare. *Practice Nursing* **8**, 29–32.

Black, P. (1997b) Practical stoma care *Nursing Standard* **11**, 49–55.

Black, P. (2000) *Holistic Stoma Care.* Ballière Tindall, London.

Bradley, M. (1997) Essential elements of ostomy care. *American Journal of Nursing* **97**, 38–45.

Bryant, R.A. (1993) Ostomy patient management. Care that engenders adaptation. *Cancer Investigations* **11**, 565–77.

Collett, K. (2002) Practical aspects of stoma management. *Nursing Standard* **17**, 45–52.

Coloplas 2nd. (1995) *Ostomy and Ostomy Patients – An Introductory Guide for Nurses.* Coloplast, Peterborough.

Davy, K. & Porrett, T. (2001) The effects of medication on bowel stomas. *Charter* **9**, 9–10.

Farbrother, M. (1993) What can I eat? *Nursing Times* **89**, 63.

Mead, J. (1994) An emphasis on practical management – discharge planning in stoma care. *Professional Nurse* **9**, 405–10.

Royal College of Nursing (2002) *RCN Standards of Care, Colorectal and Stoma Care Nursing.* RCN, London.

Taylor, P. (1995) Stomal complications. In: P. Taylor, ed. *Stoma Care in the Community: A Clinical Resource for Practitioners.* NT Books, London.

Watkins, D.K. (1987) An over view of the effects of drug therapy in those with a stoma. *Pharmaceutical Journal* **238**, 68.

Understanding Chemotherapy and Radiotherapy for the Individual with a Stoma

Anthony McGrath & Juliette Fulham

INTRODUCTION

For patients undergoing stoma formation due to a cancer, surgery will not necessarily be the only form of treatment they receive. Although surgery is the main mode of treatment for the majority of these patients – since surgical excision of the tumour offers the best chance of achieving a potential cure (Souhami & Tobias 1998) – the patient may still need to receive additional treatments with radiotherapy and/or chemo-therapy at some point.

LEARNING OBJECTIVES

By the end of this chapter, the reader should be able to:

❏ understand the rationale for chemotherapy and/or radio-therapy at different stages in the disease trajectory for patients with a cancer which has required stoma formation;
❏ have a basic understanding of how chemotherapy and radiotherapy can be effective in the treatment of a cancer;
❏ identify the most common treatment side-effects, and the impact these can have on the individual with a stoma.

THE RATIONALE FOR TREATMENT

The public often perceives radiotherapy and chemotherapy as palliative treatments, with little curative potential (Gill 1997). Chemotherapy and radiotherapy can be effective treatments at all stages of the disease trajectory – their use is not restricted to palliative treatment.

Increasingly, patients' treatment is multi-centred, e.g. surgery at a district general hospital, then chemotherapy and radiotherapy at a regional cancer centre. It is important that healthcare professionals understand the effects that chemotherapy and radiotherapy can have on patients with cancer and a stoma at all stages of their treatment journey to effectively anticipate, identify and manage any related problems.

Lack of insight into a patient's condition, and inexperience can render us wary of our ability to care for patients with complex physical and psychological needs (Corner & Wilson-Barnett 1992). This can lead to avoidance of the patient, or focusing only on those areas of care in which we feel competent (Wilkinson 1991).

As discussed in Chapter 3, a patient's cancer is 'staged' in order to determine which form(s) of treatment will most effectively cure – or limit the progress of – their disease. Treatment can therefore be classified as:

- primary – the main treatment;
- neo-adjuvant – given before surgery, aimed at reducing the size of the tumour;
- adjuvant – treatment received after the primary treatment, aimed at targeting any remaining cancer cells;
- palliative – treatment aimed at limiting the effects of disease, where a cure cannot be achieved.

To appreciate the rationale for these treatments at different stages of the patient's disease, it is necessary to understand the implications of metastatic disease (where the cancer has spread to other parts of the body), and have a basic knowledge of how chemotherapy and radiotherapy work.

METASTATIC SPREAD
Metastasis is unique to cancer and occurs where some cancerous cells separate themselves from the (primary) tumour and

Table 11.1 Common sites of spread from cancers which commonly necessitate surgery for stoma formation. From Johnson & Gross 1998

Site of primary tumour	Usual pattern of spread of disease
Bladder	Lymph nodes
	Kidneys and the genito-urinary system
	Local spread to other pelvic organs
Colon	Liver
	Lungs
	Lymph nodes
	Local spread
Ovary	Liver
	Lymph nodes
	Local spread within the pelvis
	Lung
	Bowel

travel, via blood vessels or the lymphatic system, to another site within the body, where a 'secondary' or 'metastatic' tumour grows. Table 11.1 shows common sites of spread from those cancers which commonly necessitate surgery for stoma formation (Johnson & Gross 1998). It is commonly the growth of metastatic tumour(s) at the site of a major organ (e.g. the liver) which will ultimately prove fatal for the individual with a cancer, even where the primary tumour has been removed (Ahmad & Hart 1997).

HOW CHEMOTHERAPY WORKS
Normal cells within the body are 'programmed' to replicate for a limited number of times before the cell recognises an abnormality in its DNA and cell death occurs (Souhami & Tobias 1998). Cancer cells do not have this constraint, so can continue to divide and replicate unchecked, hence the cancerous tumour develops and grows (Groenwald 1998).

Chemotherapy (or 'cytotoxic therapy') aims to inhibit, through the administration of drug(s), the process of cellular replication in cancerous cells, i.e. to bring about cell death of malignant cells. Both normal and malignant cells are affected by chemotherapy, but malignant cells are more susceptible to irreparable damage. Normal cells are more likely to be able to repair themselves (Dougherty & Bailey 2001). Chemotherapy can be referred to as:

- Single-agent chemotherapy – where one chemotherapy drug is given.
- Combination chemotherapy – where a combination of two or more drugs is administered.
- Continuous therapy – where the patient receives a continuous infusion of the chemotherapy over a fixed period of time, via a portable infusion device.
- Intermittent therapy – where the patient receives the chemotherapy drug(s) at set intervals (e.g. weekly/every three weeks).
- Cell-cycle specific – where the drug disrupts the cell at a specific phase of the cell cycle (e.g. many work by disrupting genetic codes of cells during the synthesis of DNA).
- Cell-cycle non-specific – where the drug can disrupt the cell in any phase of its cycle.

Many chemotherapy drugs are 'cell-cycle specific', yet at any given time, only a certain proportion of the tumour's cells will be at the precise phase of their cycle where the chemotherapy can be effective. It is for this reason that chemotherapy is usually given as a series of treatments at set intervals (or as a continuous infusion), rather than as a 'one-off' dose. The aim is that over a period of time, a greater proportion of cancerous cells will have been targeted. This also limits the effect of the chemotherapy on normal cells, and gives them time to repair themselves between each dose, thus lessening the severity of potential side-effects (Dougherty & Bailey 2001).

Although there are other modes of administration, chemotherapy is usually administered systemically (i.e. intravenously, via a peripherally or centrally inserted access device).

The drug circulates around the body and is therefore potentially able to target cancerous cells wherever they are within the body, i.e. both at the site of the primary tumour and at the site of any metastatic spread.

Chemotherapy is most effective in cells which are rapidly dividing (Stein 1996). The larger a tumour becomes, the greater the proportion of cells which are replicating slowly, so fewer cells are likely to be in an active phase of their cycle. Thus fewer cells are vulnerable to the effects of chemotherapy. This is why larger, more established tumours are more 'chemo-resistant', and surgery would be the primary treatment of choice (Liebman & Camp-Sorrell 1996).

Many patients will view the prospect of undergoing chemotherapy treatment with great fear and uncertainty. Indeed, many will have known somebody who has undergone chemotherapy, and even though this individual may have had a completely different form of cancer, and received a different combination of drugs, the patient may believe that they too will suffer the same side effects.

There are many chemotherapy drugs in current usage, each one having its own potential side-effects. Different types of tumour respond to different types and combinations of chemotherapeutic drugs. It is vital to explain to the patient that their oncologist (cancer specialist) will decide which chemotherapy drug(s) are best suited to them – based on the type of tumour they have, and how advanced their disease is at the time. Thus, the experiences of and side-effects in someone receiving chemotherapy for, say, lung cancer, will not be the same as for someone undergoing, say, adjuvant treatment for colorectal cancer. Moreover, not all individuals receiving the same treatment will experience the same degree of side-effects.

HOW RADIOTHERAPY WORKS
Radiotherapy (commonly referred to as 'DXT', deep x-ray therapy) aims to treat a localised (i.e. limited) area where a

cancer has occurred. Radiotherapy uses ionising radiation – where molecules and atoms are ionised to induce chemical and biological tissue changes, which cause damage to the cell's nucleus – with the aim of bringing about cell death (Faithfull 2001).

In common with chemotherapy, normal cells have a greater ability to recover from radiotherapy, compared with cancerous cells (Rice 1997). Radiotherapy is delivered in 'fractions', i.e. given in small doses, often daily, over a set period of time. This is to allow normal cells time to repair themselves between each treatment, thus limiting the side-effects. Fractionated therapy also means that hypoxic cells (those which have poor oxygen supply), which are radiotherapy-resistant, have time to re-oxygenate and redistribute themselves within the tumour, so that they are more radiotherapy-sensitive for subsequent treatments (Faithfull 2001).

Patients due to undergo radiotherapy treatment will initially undergo a session on the 'simulator'. This is the longest appointment in the patient's treatment, and it is the planning phase, where the radiologist (the radiotherapy specialist) measures and plans the specific treatment for the patient. Subsequent sessions of actual radiotherapy treatment are actually quite brief – a few minutes each.

CHEMOTHERAPY/RADIOTHERAPY AS A PRIMARY TREATMENT CHOICE

For some, chemotherapy and/or radiotherapy may be their primary mode of treatment. For instance, a patient with squamous cell carcinoma of the anus will usually undergo chemotherapy and radiotherapy with the intention of curing their disease, and thereby avoid the need for an abdominoperineal resection and formation of a permanent stoma. Some of these patients may be offered a temporary stoma for the duration of this treatment, since the peri-anal area can become very painful due to the combination of radiotherapy-induced skin damage and possible chemotherapy-induced diarrhoea. Many patients with bladder cancer will have previously undergone intra-vesical chemotherapy (where chemotherapeutic drugs are administered via a catheter directly into the bladder) in the hope of curing their cancer when it was at an earlier stage.

Similarly, some patients may have received radiotherapy as a primary treatment for more advanced (stage III) bladder cancer – in the hope of avoiding the need for a urinary stoma. Performing a total cystectomy (removal of the bladder) for these patients can present greater difficulties for the surgeons due to the local tissue and organ damage caused by the radiotherapy. In a very debilitated patient, it may be necessary for the surgeons to carry out the operation in two stages: an initial operation to perform the urinary diversion and form the urostomy/ileal conduit, and a subsequent operation (when the patient is sufficiently recovered) to remove the diseased bladder – termed a 'salvage cystectomy' (Souhami & Tobias 1998).

It is important to appreciate the needs of patients undergoing stoma surgery, for whom chemotherapy or radiotherapy as a primary mode of treatment have failed to prevent the progression of their cancer. Not only may they still be experiencing the potentially debilitating side-effects of these treatments when facing major surgery, but they also have to deal with the psychological implications that one form of treatment has already failed.

CHEMOTHERAPY/RADIOTHERAPY AS NEO-ADJUVANT TREATMENT

In the context of patients who ultimately undergo surgery for stoma formation, neo-adjuvant treatment is most commonly given to those with a rectal or ovarian tumour. Treatment pre-operatively with a course of chemotherapy and/or radiotherapy aims to reduce the risk of a recurrence of the disease postoperatively, and thereby improve overall survival rates.

The benefits to the individual, however, can vary according to age, and the stage of disease (National Institute of Clinical Excellence (NICE) 2004). Trials examining this form of treatment are on-going. Another aim of neo-adjuvant therapy can be to 'down size' the tumour, so that less extensive surgery is needed to successfully excise it (with a consequential reduction in the risk of surgical morbidity), or so that a previously unresectable tumour becomes resectable.

However, waiting times for radiotherapy are lengthy in many regions of the UK, and if this is the case, the benefits of neo-adjuvant chemo-radiation may be outweighed by the risk of disease progression while waiting to commence treatment. In such instances, the surgeon may have no choice but to proceed directly to surgery.

ADJUVANT TREATMENTS

Most patients undergoing surgery for a cancer will be scanned routinely pre-operatively to establish the extent of their disease and whether any metastatic spread has occurred. Yet, many patients who have no evidence of residual or metastatic disease following surgery will develop a recurrence of their cancer due to previously undetectable metastases. For instance, around 80% of those undergoing surgery for colorectal cancer have no evidence at surgery of residual disease or metastatic spread. However, around 50% of these will develop an ultimately fatal recurrence of their disease (NICE 2003). Adjuvant therapy is aimed at destroying any micro-metastases (metastatic deposits which may be too small to be detected by a scan or by the surgeon's naked eye).

By the time it is large enough to be detectable, a large proportion of a tumour's cells will be slowly dividing or resting (Dougherty & Bailey 2001). Yet, as already noted, chemotherapy is generally more effective on cells which are rapidly dividing. The rationale for adjuvant therapy is based on the premise that the rate of proliferation of any remaining cancer cells increases after removal of the primary tumour; hence these micro-metastases are more vulnerable to the effects of chemotherapy during the period immediately following surgery (Midgley & Kerr 2001).

When caring for patients recovering from surgery for a cancer and facing adjuvant therapy, it is therefore vital that all members of the multi-disciplinary team strive towards optimising their recovery, in order to better prepare them to face their next stage of treatment. For example, current guidelines for the treatment of colorectal cancer recommend that adjuvant therapy be instigated within six weeks of surgery (NICE 2003). The onset of treatment can be delayed for patients who have a postoperative wound infection, or delayed wound healing. Indeed, if the patient is considered to be too debilitated, they may be deemed unfit for adjuvant treatment.

Chemotherapy/radiotherapy as a palliative treatment

Treatment is given in this context for the following reasons:

- to treat residual disease (where it has not been possible to surgically excise the entire tumour due to the extent of its spread, or where it is known that metastatic spread has already occurred);
- to treat a recurrence of the disease (where a complete surgical excision of the recurrent tumour is not possible);
- for an unresectable tumour (where the spread of the tumour may be so extensive that surgical excision is impossible), e.g. in advanced ovarian cancer, where a palliative colostomy may have already been created to resolve a bowel obstruction;
- to achieve palliation or relief from symptoms caused by an advanced cancer.

Traditional perceptions of the 'success' of treatments (i.e. overall survival rates) are changing, and, particularly in the context of palliative therapies, the effect of treatment on quality of life versus improved survival is increasingly considered (McPhail 1999).

EFFECTS OF PREVIOUS TREATMENT NECESSITATING STOMA FORMATION

For some, the effects of previous treatments may *cause* the need for a stoma. For instance, patients who have previously received pelvic radiotherapy may experience radiotherapy-induced proctitis (where the mucosa of the rectum bleeds, becomes ulcerated or ischaemic or a fistula develops) (Jones 1999), which, if the symptoms are severe, may require permanent or temporary stoma formation. Modern advances in radiotherapy now mean that damage to surrounding tissue and organs is limited as much as possible, and hopefully this reason for stoma formation will become increasingly uncommon.

SIDE-EFFECTS OF TREATMENT

The most commonly experienced side-effects of chemotherapy and radiotherapy will be discussed here. While individuals with or without a stoma can potentially experience all of these, it is important to appreciate how these problems can uniquely affect those who have undergone stoma surgery.

As healthcare professionals, it is vital to monitor patients for potential side-effects at each encounter and to encourage them to inform their healthcare team promptly if any side-effects do occur. Some patients may believe these side-effects are an inevitable outcome of treatment which they are expected to endure, and some may be reluctant to alert us to any side-effects, for fear that their treatment may be halted or reduced. It is important to reassure them that early identification and treatment of any side-effects is much less likely to result in a curtailment of their treatment than if the side-effects remain untreated and become more severe.

Common side-effects and problems associated with radiotherapy

Fatigue

This can occur both during and after treatment. Faithfull (2001) discussed how the incidence of fatigue among patients undergoing radiotherapy was found to range from 65% to 100%. The presence of fatigue is not dose limiting. Knowledge is limited about why radiotherapy induces fatigue. It is suggested that an accumulation of metabolites from cell destruction and the increased demands upon the body for repair of damaged cells may be causes (Faithfull 2001). There is limited research examining effective interventions.

It should be considered that those patients who have received neo-adjuvant radiotherapy prior to surgery are still likely to be experiencing radiotherapy-induced fatigue at the time they undergo their surgery. Staff involved in the care of these patients should consider the impact this can have upon their postoperative recovery.

Skin damage

Skin reactions to radiotherapy are caused by radiobiological damage to cells within the dermis and epidermis (Korinko & Yurick 1997). Skin damage can be classified as:

- Erythema – Skin feels dry, warm and red; occurs within two to three weeks of radiotherapy being started; resolves within two to three weeks of therapy finishing.
- Dry desquamation – pruritus and dry, peeling skin are present; can occur within two to three weeks of radiotherapy being started.
- Moist desquamation – skin blisters and sloughs off, exposing the dermis; serous fluid oozes from the damaged area.
- Necrosis – this rarely occurs (Faithfull 2001).

Skin folds (e.g. the perineal area) are more likely to sustain damage, as are areas which have had recent surgery (as is the case for patients who have undergone an abdominoperineal resection for a rectal cancer, who may go on to receive adjuvant radiotherapy). Similarly, patients undergoing neo-adjuvant radiotherapy and subsequent abdominoperineal resection can experience delayed healing to their perineal wound due to radiotherapy-induced skin damage. Moreover, combined therapy (i.e. radiotherapy and chemotherapy) can make the skin more vulnerable to damage.

Preventative measures

Patients should be advised that they may wash the skin within the treatment area. Moisturising creams should be applied, although alcohol and petroleum-based creams and those containing lanolin should be avoided (Korinko & Yurick 1997). Cream should not be applied within two hours prior to treatment, and patients should avoid a build-up of cream (this can be prevented by washing the area). Loose, cotton clothing should be worn over the treatment area, and exposure to the sun should be avoided.

Treatment when skin damage has occurred

Topical steroids can be useful for pruritus (itching) associated with dry desquamation, but prolonged use of these should be avoided, since this could affect skin thickness. For areas of moist desquamation, hydrogel dressings (e.g. Geliperm) may be appropriate. If the volume of exudate from the area is moderate/heavy, an alginate dressing (e.g. Sorbsan/Aquacel) may be required. Hydrocolloid sheets can also be effective (Faithfull 2001).

When selecting a dressing to treat an affected area, it should be considered that if treatment is on-going, dressings within the treatment field may need to be removed for each treatment. Tapes or film dressings should be avoided to secure the primary dressing – removal of these may cause skin damage (Faithfull 2001).

Sexuality

Radiotherapy can affect sexual functioning, physically or psychologically. Patients with a stoma undergoing treatment have already experienced a major alteration in their body image, and this, combined with radiotherapy and/or chemotherapy-induced fatigue can cause a loss of libido. Additionally, those undergoing treatment for gynaecological cancers can experience early menopause, loss of fertility or vaginal fibrosis (which can also be experienced by women who have undergone an abdominoperineal resection). In men, radiotherapy to the perineum or pelvis can cause erectile dysfunction.

Gastrointestinal disturbances (radiotherapy enteritis)

For patients undergoing abdominal or pelvic radiotherapy, other organs within the field can sustain long- or short-term damage, notably the small intestine and colon. In the short term this can cause nausea, diarrhoea, pain, tenesmus (a persistent urge to defecate) and abdominal cramps (Faithfull 2001). Unresolved nausea will result in anorexia, and reduced nutritional intake. Uncontrolled persistent diarrhoea will result in malabsorption of essential nutrients, resulting in malnutrition as well as potential dehydration.

Epithelial cells in intestinal mucosa divide rapidly and therefore are particularly easily damaged by radiotherapy (Rice 1997). Acute damage resolves once treatment is completed, but secondary damage can occur months or years after treatment, causing rectal bleeding, fistula formation, ulceration to the rectum and colon, strictures, diarrhoea, obstruction and ulceration to the small intestine (Faithfull 2001).

Management of acute damage

Patients affected by acute damage will require regular monitoring of their weight and nutritional intake. Ileostomists are particularly vulnerable to the effects of radiotherapy enteritis and should be advised to be alert for signs of dehydration, since their condition could deteriorate rapidly if symptoms remain uncontrolled. Colostomists experiencing diarrhoea will require a supply of drainable bags. The benefit of dietary intervention is disputed, but a low-fat, low-residue diet may be suggested (Faithfull 2001). Anti-diarrhoeals such as loperamide or codeine phosphate may be prescribed.

Management of long-term damage
Surgical intervention may be necessary, and (as discussed earlier in this chapter) for some, this is why stoma surgery is actually required.

Positioning required for treatment

The position the patient needs to adopt for radiotherapy treatment to be administered may present problems for the individual with a stoma. For instance, some patients undergoing radiotherapy may need to lie on their front, which means they will need to ensure their bag is emptied immediately prior to each treatment, and that they have a securely fitting appliance, if leaks are to be prevented. Stoma patients should be advised to always ensure they bring spare bags with them. The patient's stoma bag (and its contents if a transparent appliance is being used, which is particularly likely to be the case for new ostomists who may still find positioning their bag properly difficult) may be visible during the treatment. This may be a source of great concern to the patient.

Common side-effects and problems associated with chemotherapy

This section will focus on short- and long-term side-effects to chemotherapy, since immediate side-effects (occurring shortly after administration of the drug(s) begins) would generally occur while the patient is in the chemotherapy unit/cancer centre receiving their treatment. It is not possible within the limits of this chapter to list all chemotherapeutic drugs an individual with cancer and a stoma could potentially receive. However, Table 11.2 lists the most commonly used

Table 11.2 Commonly used chemotherapy drugs for patients with colorectal, ovarian or bladder cancer. From www.cancerhelp.org.uk and www.cancerbacup.org.uk

Site of primary tumour	Commonly used chemotherapy agents	Common side-effects
Colorectal	5-fluorouracil (can be given orally in tablet form when it is known as capecitabine (brand name Xeloda))	Palmar-plantar syndrome, gastrointestinal disturbances, neutropenia, peripheral neuropathy, sometimes hair thinning, oral mucositis
	Mitomycin C	Neutropenia, anaemia, reduced platelets, infertility, reduced appetite
	Oxaliplatin	Peripheral neuropathy, nausea and vomiting, neutropenia, anaemia, reduced platelets, diarrhoea, oral mucositis, infertility
	Irinotecan	Diarrhoea (this can become severe, and patients will be given specific instructions), nausea and vomiting, reduced appetite, neutropenia, anaemia, reduced platelets, alopecia or hair thinning
Ovarian	Carboplatin	Neutropenia, anaemia, reduced platelets, nausea and vomiting, fatigue, reduced appetite
	Paclitaxel (Taxol)	Neutropenia, anaemia, reduced platelets, oral mucositis, diarrhoea, alopecia, skin rashes, fatigue, peripheral neuropathy, nausea and vomiting, muscular and joint pain, headaches, allergic reaction

Bladder		
	Methotrexate	Neutropenia, anaemia, reduced platelets, oral mucositis, diarrhoea, changes in taste, fatigue, alopecia/hair thinning, gritty eyes
	Vinblastine	Neutropenia, anaemia, reduced platelets, hair thinning (occasional alopecia), nausea, oral mucositis, infertility, occasional peripheral neuropathy
	Doxorubicin (Adriamycin)	Neutropenia, anaemia, reduced platelets, nausea and vomiting, alopecia, oral mucositis, discoloured urine, increased lacrimation, sensitivity to sun, infertility
	Cisplatin	Nausea and vomiting, slight deafness, infertility, renal failure, neutropenia, anaemia, reduced platelets
	Gemcitabine	Neutropenia, anaemia, reduced platelets, nausea and vomiting, reduced appetite, impaired renal and liver function, fluid retention, skin rashes, fatigue

chemotherapeutic drugs for patients with colorectal, ovarian or bladder cancer.

Fatigue

Although (in common with radiotherapy) the exact mechanism that causes fatigue in patients receiving chemotherapy is not fully understood, the majority of patients undergoing chemotherapy experience this to varying degrees. Achieving adequate rest and adopting strategies to enable patients to cope with the effects of chemotherapy-induced fatigue are of paramount importance. Its presence is not usually dose limiting.

Gastrointestinal disturbances (nausea and vomiting, diarrhoea and constipation)

The occurrence of gastrointestinal disturbances due to chemotherapy is, inevitably, a distressing and debilitating symptom for all patients. In patients who have also undergone stoma formation, side-effects such as diarrhoea can lead to additional problems in their stoma management with fear of appliance leaks, or discomfort from excoriated skin.

The nutritional status of patients who have recently undergone surgery for cancer is often sub-optimal before chemotherapy commences and can be further reduced by treatment-induced damage to the gastrointestinal tract. The presence of these side-effects can limit the patient's social activities and interactions, which may already have been curtailed due to their reaction to stoma formation.

Nausea and vomiting

Chemotherapy drugs vary in the degree of nausea and vomiting they may induce. Patients receiving those drugs which are known to cause nausea and vomiting beyond the acute phase will (as well as receiving anti-emetics at the time of administration) be given a supply of oral anti-emetics to take at home for a short period following treatment.

Occasionally, individuals find these ineffective and experience severe nausea and vomiting. It is vital that their oncology team is made aware of this, so that other anti-emetics (or alternative modes of administration) can be tried. They may even require a continuous infusion of anti-emetics to control the problem for subsequent cycles of chemotherapy.

Patients with ileostomies are particularly vulnerable to the effects of prolonged vomiting and can quickly become dehydrated with deranged fluid and electrolyte levels. Prompt medical intervention is vital if a rapid deterioration in their condition is to be prevented.

Patients experiencing ongoing nausea and vomiting in the days following administration of chemotherapy may benefit from adjusting their meal patterns. Eating 'little and often', avoiding fatty foods and eating cold meals (to avoid the odours from cooking) are all useful strategies (Dougherty & Bailey 2001).

Diarrhoea

The cells which line the intestine replicate rapidly (Rice 1997). When the level of normal cell replication is reduced, due to the effects of chemotherapy, the epithelial lining of the bowel becomes inflamed and swollen, and the villi and microvilli lining the bowel atrophy, which decreases the absorptive surface of the bowel. This causes a more rapid gut transit time, and malabsorption of essential nutrients, resulting in diarrhoea (Dougherty & Bailey 2001). It is a common side-effect of 5-fluorouracil (and its oral equivalents) – the chemotherapeutic agent most commonly given to treat patients with a colorectal cancer.

It should be noted that severe diarrhoea is a known side-effect of irinotecan (Ferns 2003), a drug commonly used in the treatment of advanced colorectal cancer. Patients receiving this drug will have received specific instructions regarding the management of this, including at what stage to seek urgent medical treatment and will have been provided with a supply of anti-diarrhoeal medication.

It is important to establish a 'base-line', i.e. the patient's normal pattern of elimination, in order to determine the severity of symptoms. Patients with a stoma – ileostomists in particular – may find it difficult to identify diarrhoea, due to their altered pattern of elimination. They should be encouraged to establish whether the frequency of emptying/changing their appliance has increased, or if their output has become looser or watery.

It is vital that colostomists experiencing diarrhoea are given a supply of drainable appliances to use while any diarrhoea persists; a closed pouch will fill up with loose stool very quickly, and will require repeated changes causing the patient's skin to become sore. Indeed, any patient with a newly formed colostomy who is expected to undergo chemotherapy in the future should be provided with a supply of drainable, as well as closed, bags on discharge from hospital, and should be aware of how to obtain further supplies.

As with radiation enteritis, ileostomists can rapidly become acutely unwell if diarrhoea persists. They should understand the need to maintain an adequate intake of food and fluids, and to seek immediate medical advice if their side-effects from chemotherapy prevent them from doing so. They should be made aware of the signs and symptoms of dehydration. For inpatients, accurate maintenance of fluid balance records and frequent monitoring of nutritional intake and nutritional status are vital.

Patients experiencing diarrhoea should be encouraged to eat low-residue, high-protein, high-calorie foods, and avoid fatty or high-fibre foods while the diarrhoea persists to promote absorption of nutrients. Anti-diarrhoeal drugs (such as loperamide) will often be prescribed. It should be noted that ileostomists will require this in a suspension, since capsules or tablets may not be properly absorbed, due to their reduced gut transit time. The usual advice is to take a dose of loperamide after each episode of diarrhoea (up to a maximum of four times per day), but this will be impossible for an ileostomist to determine. Consequently, ileostomists should also be advised to take the medication around an hour *before* meals, in order to slow down the gut transit time, so that the subsequent meal is better absorbed (Black 1985).

Constipation
Conversely, constipation can be a side-effect of some chemotherapy drugs (including 5-fluorouracil and vinblastine). Encouraging a high-fibre diet and adequate fluid intake, in conjunction with prescribed aperients and stool softeners is necessary. Enemas and suppositories will, of course, be of no benefit to the ostomist.

Mucositis/stomatitis
Chemotherapeutic drugs known to cause this problem include 5-fluorouracil, methotrexate, doxorubicin, bleomycin and mitomycin C. This is a potentially dose-limiting side-effect where the mucous membranes of all areas of the mouth (including the lips) and the pharynx become acutely inflamed and ulcerated (Dougherty & Bailey 2001). It occurs due to chemotherapy-induced cell damage, or damage to blood cells (discussed below) where impaired resistance to infection and increased likelihood of bleeding in the gastrointestinal tract can occur. The cells within the mucosal membranes renew themselves every 10–14 days, so symptoms can manifest themselves as early as three days after administration of chemotherapy (Dougherty & Bailey 2001).

Pre-disposing factors include impaired nutritional status, poor dental hygiene and pre-existing oral health, in addition to the type and dose of the chemotherapy agent(s) (Focazio 1997).

If mucositis becomes severe and where infection, sloughing or ulceration have occurred the patient may find it very difficult to eat and drink. Again, ileostomists are at particular risk of acute dehydration if symptoms cause them to limit their intake. More minor manifestations are reduced production of saliva, inflammation and a burning sensation when eating spicy or acidic foods.

A regular oral assessment should be performed routinely on all patients undergoing chemotherapy. Patients should be advised to pay close attention to their oral hygiene throughout treatment, using a soft toothbrush (to avoid trauma to oral tissue). Anti-bacterial mouthwashes and anti-fungal preparations may be prescribed, together with topical preparations or emollients to apply to cracked lips. The patient may need to adjust their diet – bland foods, with a softer consistency may be better tolerated (Dougherty & Bailey 2001). For those with severe symptoms, nutritional support (with appropriate intervention from a dietitian) may be required.

Chemotherapy can also affect the condition of the stoma during treatment. The stoma can become oedematous and appear inflamed. Since the stoma contains no nerves, this cannot cause the patient any pain, but they should be advised to be alert for changes in the shape and size of their stoma and to adjust the size of the hole in their appliance accordingly.

Suppression of bone marrow (myelosuppression): neutropenia, thrombocytopenia and anaemia

Stem cells in bone marrow divide rapidly, and are affected by most chemotherapeutic drugs. These side-effects can be dose limiting, and can cause potentially fatal complications, notably sepsis or haemorrhage (Dougherty & Bailey 2001).

Neutropenia (reduction in the volume of white blood cells)
White blood cells (leucocytes) divide every six to eight hours, so are affected the soonest by chemotherapy-induced cell damage. A decreased neutrophil count renders a patient more vulnerable to infection. Treatment with antibiotics or anti-fungal drugs, and protective isolation may be required.

Subsequent chemotherapy cycles may need to be reduced, delayed or even terminated. Staphylococcal, pseudomonal and fungal infections are those most commonly experienced (Dougherty & Bailey 2001).

The earliest sign of infection is usually pyrexia, although it should be noted that in a neutropenic patient normal inflammatory response may be impaired, so that other, usually obvious, signs of infection (e.g. pus or inflammation at an infected cannula site) may not be apparent.

Patients should be encouraged to avoid crowds, or people with known infections, when their neutrophil counts are low, pay close attention to personal and oral hygiene and avoid damaging the integrity of skin and mucous membranes (including at the stoma site), for example by using a soft toothbrush and an electric razor rather than a 'wet shave'. Invasive medical procedures (e.g. intramuscular injections) should, therefore, only be performed where absolutely necessary.

Specialised drugs (known as haematopoietic growth factors) are available which can increase the volume of neutrophils. Their effectiveness in limiting the severity of neutropenia means their use is becoming more widespread.

Thrombocytopenia (reduction in the volume of platelets)
Platelets divide every seven to ten days. A reduced platelet count means the patient is at greater risk of bleeding or bruising. Platelet transfusions may be required. Patients with a stoma may notice increased bleeding at the stoma site when cleaning their stoma. For those patients on warfarin, there is a greater risk that clotting will become deranged. They need frequent INR (international normalised ratio) checks.

Anaemia
Red blood cells divide approximately every 120 days. This means that severe chemotherapy-induced anaemia is less

common, and occurs much later in treatment. Blood transfusions may be necessary.

Palmar-plantar erythrodyaesthesia and peripheral neuropathy

Palmar-plantar syndrome (or 'hand/foot syndrome') is a side effect of 5-fluorouracil (the most commonly used chemotherapy drug for colorectal cancer) and its oral equivalents. The palms of the hands and the soles of the feet become swollen and painful, with cracked, dry and flaky skin. Regular application of a moisturiser (e.g. Diprobase) is a useful preventive and treatment measure. If plantar-palmar syndrome occurs, the patient will usually be prescribed pyridoxine (vitamin B) to help alleviate symptoms.

Peripheral neuropathy ('pins and needles' and numbness in the hands and feet) is a side-effect associated with oxaliplatin (commonly used for advanced colorectal cancer) and some other chemotherapeutic agents. It can take several months to resolve.

Both these side-effects can result in impaired manual dexterity, which may mean the patient with a stoma finds appliance changes or emptying their bag more difficult. It may be necessary to switch to a different appliance if the patient is experiencing difficulties with their current one.

Changes to body image: alopecia, weight loss and cancer cachexia

Chemotherapy, radiotherapy and the effects of progressive disease can have further effects on a patient's body-image, at a time when surgery for stoma formation may have already profoundly altered their self-image. Alopecia, hair thinning and weight loss are common side effects of treatment, while weight loss and cancer cachexia are common manifestations of progressive disease. These visible effects can serve as another reminder to the patient and those around them of their disease and further undermine an individual's self esteem.

For patients with a diagnosis of cancer who have undergone surgery resulting in stoma formation, it is important for healthcare professionals to appreciate the physical and psychological burdens their treatment places on them. They are often expected to undergo chemotherapy and/or radiotherapy at a time when they are still dealing with the psychological effects of being diagnosed with a potentially life-limiting disease, experiencing a major alteration in their body image, meeting the physical and practical demands of recovering from surgery (or facing the prospect of further surgery) and adjusting to caring for their stoma. Sensitive and informed care at all stages of their treatment journey is vital to help them cope with the challenges their disease and its treatment impose upon them.

SELF-EVALUATION QUESTIONS AND ANSWERS

Questions

1. What is the main mode of curative treatment for individuals with a colorectal cancer?
   A. Chemotherapy
   B. Radiotherapy
   C. Surgery
   D. Complementary therapies

2. When is adjuvant chemotherapy for colorectal cancer given?
   A. Pre-operatively
   B. After removal of the bladder
   C. Postoperatively
   D. During the end stages of disease

3. What percentage of patients with colorectal cancer undergoing surgery have no evidence of metastatic spread at the time of surgery?
   A. 50%
   B. 80%
   C. 30%
   D. 10%

4. Which of the following foods/drinks would be suitable for someone experiencing oral mucositis?
   A. Salt and vinegar crisps
   B. Wine
   C. Ice cream
   D. Oranges

5. Name three common side-effects associated with radiotherapy.

6. Name the four types of skin damage that can occur as a result of radiotherapy.

7. Along with nausea and vomiting, what other debilitating gastrointestinal symptom could occur for patients with an ileostomy receiving chemotherapy that would make managing their stoma difficult?

8. Why is chemotherapy less effective on large, established tumours (i.e. the size they have reached by the time they are usually clinically detectable)?

9. Why is it a good idea for anyone undergoing chemotherapy to have a thermometer available at home?

10. What type of product should patients with a colostomy always be provided with before they start their chemotherapy?

Answers

1. A. Surgery is the only form of treatment which really offers the chance of achieving a cure.

2. C. Postoperatively, with the aim of eradicating any micro-metastases.

3. B. 80% – although half of these will experience a recurrence of their cancer, even though there was no evidence of residual disease after their surgery.

4. Ice cream – the others would cause pain and a 'burning' sensation for someone experiencing mucositis. Bland, soft foods are often best tolerated.

5. Fatigue, skin damage, gastrointestinal disturbances (nausea and vomiting and diarrhoea).

6. Erythema, dry desquamation, moist desquamation and necrosis.

7. Diarrhoea. This could cause an ileostomist to become acutely unwell very quickly, if they are unable to replace the fluids and electrolytes lost through their stoma and resolve the diarrhoea.

8. Chemotherapy is most effective in cells which are rapidly dividing. By the time it is large enough to be detected, a large proportion of cells in a tumour will be replicating slowly. Chemotherapy will not be effective on these cells, therefore will not succeed in shrinking the tumour appreciably. This is why surgery is the primary treatment of choice for 'solid tumours', offering the best chance of a cure.

9. A raised temperature is one of the first signs of infection. Infection is common among patients receiving chemotherapy who become neutropenic (reduced level of white blood cells). Severe neutropenia, or infection, will require medical intervention.

10. Drainable bags. If they experience chemotherapy-induced diarrhoea, their stoma bags will fill up quickly and it is impractical to change a closed bag frequently. This will also cause the peri-stomal skin to become sore, so switching to drainable bags while the diarrhoea persists is best.

REFERENCES

Ahmad, A. & Hart, I. (1997) Mechanisms of metastasis. *Critical Reviews in Oncology-Haematology* **26**, 163–73.

Black, P. (1985) Stoma care: drugs and diet. *Nursing Mirror* **161**, 26–8.

Corner, J. & Wilson-Barnett, J. (1992) The newly registered nurse and the cancer patient: an educational evaluation. *International Journal of Nursing Studies* **29**, 177–90.

Dougherty, L. & Bailey, C. (2001) Chemotherapy. In: J. Corner & C. Bailey, eds. *Cancer Nursing. Care in Context*, pp. 179–221. Blackwell Science, Oxford.

Faithfull, S. (2001) Radiotherapy. In: J. Corner & C. Bailey, eds. *Cancer Nursing. Care in Context*, pp. 222–61. Blackwell Science, Oxford.

Ferns, H. (2003) Campto effective and flexible chemotherapy for advanced colorectal cancer. *International Journal of Palliative Nursing* **9**, 290–7.

Focazio, B. (1997) Mucositis. *American Journal of Nursing* **97**, 48–9.

Gill, O. (1997) The challenge of cancer: improving essential nursing skills. *Nursing Standard* **11**, 5–25.

Groenwald, S. (1998) The behaviour of malignancies. In: B. Johnson & J. Cross, eds. *Handbook of Oncology Nursing*, 3rd edn, pp. 3–20. Jones & Bartlett Publishers, Massachusetts.

Johnson, B. & Gross, J. (1998) *Handbook of Oncology Nursing*, 3rd edn. Jones & Bartlett Publishers, Massachusetts.

Jones, D.J. (1999) Lower gastrointestinal haemorrhage. In: D.J. Jones, ed. *ABC of Colorectal Diseases*, pp. 17–200. BMJ Publishing Group, London.

Korinko, A. & Yurick, A. (1997) Maintaining skin integrity during radiation therapy. *American Journal of Nursing* **97**, 40–4.

Liebman, M. & Camp-Sorrell, D. (1996) *Multi-Modal Therapy in Oncology Nursing*. Mosby Year-book Inc., Missouri.

Midgley, R.S.J. & Kerr, D.J. (2001) Adjuvant therapy. In: D.J. Jones & M.H. Irving, eds. *ABC of Colorectal Cancer*, pp. 15–18. BMJ Publishing Group, London.

McPhail, G. (1999) Chemotherapy in palliative cancer care: changing perspectives. *International Journal of Palliative Nursing* **5**, 81–6.

National Institute for Clinical Excellence (NICE) (2003) *Improving Outcomes in Colorectal Cancer. Manual Update 3c*. Department of Health, London.

National Institute for Clinical Excellence (NICE) (2004) *Guidance for Commissioning Cancer Services. Improving Outcomes in Colorectal Cancers. Research Evidence for the Manual Update*. Department of Health, London.

Rice, A.M. (1997) An introduction to radiotherapy. *Nursing Standard* **12**, 49–56.

Souhami, R. & Tobias, J. (1998) *Cancer and Its Management*. Blackwell Science, Oxford.

Stein, P. (1996) Chemotherapy. In: V. Tschudin, ed. *Nursing The Patient with Cancer*, 2nd edn, pp. 78–95. Prentice Hall International (UK) Ltd., Hertfordshire.

Wilkinson, S. (1991) Factors which influence how nurses communicate with cancer patients. *Journal of Advanced Nursing* **16**, 677–88.

Psychological Issues in Stoma Care

12

Julia Williams

LEARNING OBJECTIVES

By the end of this chapter the reader will be able to:

❏ discuss the psychological problems faced by patients undergoing stoma formation;
❏ understand the issues that surround body image;
❏ identify the role of the nurse in exploring these issues with the patient.

INTRODUCTION

People who undergo stoma surgery must not only contend with the immediate physical changes that the surgery brings about but must also adjust to the psychological impact of stoma formation. Indeed the whole experience of having a gastrointestinal illness resulting in stoma surgery represents a major change in a patient's life. The patient is in a position where they have to cope with a complex 'roller-coaster' of emotional, social and physical problems associated with the newly formed stoma. The anxieties faced will include feelings of alteration in their body image, function and control of stoma as well as restrictions within their current lifestyle and activity, all of which have the potential to impinge on sexual function. This chapter will explore the psychological impact of stoma surgery such as changes in body image, self-concept and sexual well-being and will explore ways in which we as nurses can assist the patient through this period of adaptation.

Over the years several quality of life studies (Kelman & Minkler 1989; Wade 1989; Pieper & Mikols 1996; Nugent *et al.*

1999) have been undertaken in order to determine the anxieties felt by new stoma patients so that healthcare professionals can offer a greater understanding into this group of patients' needs. Many of the concerns which patients with stomas have are often discussed in terms of body image problems; therefore the anxieties and fears of many stoma patients include, noise, odour, leakage, visibility of appliance and perceived attractiveness to others. While these anxieties are mainly practicalities of stoma care management, studies suggest that these issues contribute to the psychological adjustment and adaptation of the patient (Wade 1989).

Patients more likely to experience difficulties in psychological adjustment include those who have a reported history of psychological problems, those who express dissatisfaction with pre-operative information and those expressing negative thoughts of stoma surgery and its impact (White 1998). It is important to remember that some patients will react with shock and disgust at the thought of having a stoma as this type of surgery has a profound effect on the mind as well as the body (Salter 1997). With this in mind it is not uncommon for patients with newly formed stomas to express feelings of degradation, isolation, stigma, social restriction and mutilation (Klopp 1990).

BODY IMAGE

The way we see ourselves is an important part of our everyday lives. If there is a sudden alteration in this picture it can have psychological implications for our behaviour. Price (1990) describes body image as 'the picture we form in our minds of how our body looks and the experience we have of how our body feels, behaves and conforms to commands we give it. . . . our thoughts are based upon the reality of our body as it changes and ages and we are influenced by social, cultural and personal norms'. When an individual becomes ill he becomes far more aware of his body. If the illness also results in changes to body image then psychological difficulties may occur while adapting to the alteration (Price 1990).

In the literature reviewed, it is well recognised that patients undergoing stoma formation face permanent changes to their body image, lifestyle and sexuality (Borwell 1999; Weerakoon 2001; Salter 2002; Virgin-Elliston 2003). It has been suggested that when a stoma is raised, an immense price is paid for cure, in terms of both the physical and the psychological impact (Devlin *et al.* 1971). Stoma patients soon become aware of their change in body image, in some instances there is a painful perineal wound which reminds them they no longer have a rectum, while a bright pink 'attachment' has appeared on their abdomen encased in a plastic stoma bag as an introduction to their new way of defaecating. Having to wear an external appliance is seen as one of the main disadvantages of stoma formation, as when function occurs, it is noisy, odorous, warm against the skin and beyond their control and has the potential to lead to a profound change in feelings of body image and sexuality.

According to Newell (1991) the concept of body image is poorly defined but should include neurological, sociological and psychological aspects while Price (1990) suggests inclusion of genetics, socialisation, culture, race, fashion, the media and health education. Cohen (1991) suggests that body attributes affecting body image should also include total body size, proportion of body parts, colouration, sexuality, texture of skin and facial features. Although the literature implies body image is extremely complex it can be simply defined as 'the way we see ourselves and the way we feel about how others see us' (Salter 1997). It is important to note that body image can be as complex as an individual wishes and never remains static.

Body image is recognised as being intrinsically linked to the notions of self-concept, self-esteem and self-worth from which a person functions (Price 1990). Wassner (1992) accepts that if people are happy with their physical appearance they are more likely to experience positive feelings of self-esteem whereas in contrast, Burnard and Morrison (1990) suggest that someone who is unhappy with their appearance will experience negative feelings regarding themselves.

Change in physical appearance may make individuals feel less attractive. These feelings can lead to insecurity, lack of confidence and being out of control, which in turn can be a threat to existing relationships and friendships. Body image is related to the concept of wholeness and any loss of a body part can lead to an alteration thus affecting the individual's picture of their self.

Schain (1980; cited in Borwell 1999) suggests that self-concept consists of four components, namely:

- the body self – physical function and body image;
- the interpersonal self – sexual and psychosocial interaction;
- the achievement self – individual status and function;
- the identification self – beliefs, attitudes and values.

As individuals we are all unique, and these four areas will differ and thus will have an influence on a person's acceptance of body image, for example, the way we view ourselves in relation to others and how we communicate that to one another. The appearance of other people can therefore influence how an individual feels and sees themselves and will ultimately affect their perception of others. Beliefs, attitudes and values towards the concepts of body image are developed from early childhood and are swayed primarily by our up-bringing and influenced by our parents, friends, peers and attitudes within society.

Price (1990) illustrates this as a framework exploring aspects of the patient's body reality, body ideal and body presentation. This allows the nurse practitioner to not only assess the patient's needs with regard to the felt alteration in body image but also allows the practitioner to reflect on the adaptation and progress the patient is making during the period of rehabilitation. Body reality refers to how the body really is, whether it is tall, short, fat, or thin. Body ideal is measured constantly against an ideal of what we think the body should look like and how it should act while body presentation relates to how the body is presented to the outside world. Our body image not only includes how we feel about ourselves but also the attitudes of others. An imbalance in any given area is likely to result in an alteration in body image. The severity of this depends on two factors: the amount of support surrounding the individual and personal coping strategies.

Salter (2002) also suggests that the degree of altered body image felt by the individual not only depends upon which body part is affected but also the extent and implications of the physical alteration. Batchelor *et al.* (1991) support this by suggesting body image concern can affect how patients feel about themselves and their loved ones and can ultimately influence their quality of life.

Patients with newly formed stomas undoubtedly face changes in their appearance but they also experience loss of control over elimination which for a number of patients can be most disturbing. The fear of the stoma being detected, whether it can be smelt or heard, i.e. the passage of wind or rustle of the bag, has been expressed by patients in several studies (Church 1986; Wade 1989; Salter 2002). We are taught from an early age that being incontinent is socially unacceptable so this fear and loss of control delivers a severe blow to the self-esteem and gives rise to fears of rejection by friends and of being ostracised by society.

Illness or disability may bring about great emotional pressures and consequently people need to be able to think about their situation, sometimes in privacy and sometimes with those close to them or with healthcare professionals. The planning and implementation of care for a patient with a newly formed stoma is very important, as the effects of stoma surgery have the potential to alienate patients from social activity so that they become reclusive in nature and create elements of depression. The loss of part of their internal organs and the creation of an external one is a loss that needs to be mourned and the patient may well go through the various stages of grief (Salter 2002).

SEXUAL WELL-BEING

Human beings have the need for sexual expression throughout life despite disabilities and major illness. Sexuality encompasses much more than physical acts of sexual expression and involves the totality of being human. Sexuality involves biological, psychological and social aspects and a person's self-image, feelings and relationships with others affect sexual behaviours (Sprunk and Alteneder 2000). The World Health Organization (1975) offers three basic elements of sexual well-being:

- The capacity to enjoy and control sexual and reproductive behaviour in accordance with social and personal ethics.
- Freedom from fear, shame, guilt, misconceptions and other psychological factors that inhibit the sexual response and impair sexual relationships.
- Freedom from organic disorders, disease and deficiencies that may interfere with either sexual or reproductive function or both.

However, it must be remembered that expressing sexuality is much more than sexual intercourse alone, as ultimately it is a human contact, comfort and security, a measure of self-worth providing cohesion in a relationship (Borwell 1997). Therefore the effect of stoma formation in both men and women can be described as indirect because more often than not the issues are related to the stoma's position on the abdomen and its lack of control. In some instances sexual function in patients with stomas is reported to be unchanged or in fact slightly improved (Weerakoon 2001). What appears to concern patients most is the issue of when and how to disclose they have a stoma to others without the fear of being rejected by individuals who are close to them and/or have an influence on them.

Male sexual dysfunction

Surgery that results in stoma formation may result in damage to the nerves that control ejaculation and erection and cause altered sexual function in men. The amount of nerve damage depends on the location and degree of ligation during surgery, for example the risk of impotence is extremely high in men who have undergone radical cystectomy. Studies show that that approximately 90% of men have reported impotence following such surgery for bladder cancer (Andersen 1993); this is because the urethra and prostate are frequently removed and the erectile nerve ultimately becomes damaged.

Impotence is the inability to have or sustain an erection long enough for satisfactory intercourse and can prove to be a significant problem for men. Sexual dysfunction also may take the form of retrograde ejaculation or dry orgasms. In this instance the bladder neck fails to close properly during orgasm resulting in semen entering the bladder rather than being forced out through the urethra. Sterility or an inability to produce sperm also may be a result of stoma surgery (Young-McCaughan 1999), and for men who engage in anal intercourse the loss of the rectum can remove a major source of pleasure (Salter 2002).

Female sexual dysfunction

The most common sexual dysfunction reported by women with stomas is dyspareunia or painful intercourse (Sprunk and Alteneder 2000). Scar tissue from the pelvic operation may create bands around the vagina thus causing constriction or tightness. The pelvic surgery also results in the drying of the vagina's natural lubrication, and the consequence of both constriction and vaginal dryness is pain from friction during sexual intercourse. Lack of vaginal lubrication may also be a result of the menopause or removal of ovaries resulting in a decrease oestrogen production (Golis 1996).

If the rectum has been removed, for example, in a panproctocolectomy resulting in permanent ileostomy, the angle of the vagina will change and so too will penetration on intercourse. This may also result in orgasm being more difficult to achieve. The uterus may also change position and result in difficulties of infertility (Salter 2002). In the advent of pregnancy difficulties may arise, including stomal complications such as stoma prolapse and/or bowel obstruction.

IMPLICATIONS FOR NURSING CARE

Some patients who are about to undergo stoma surgery may not have heard of the operation before or may have found information via the internet and be filled with horror. Others just do not want to discuss the subject until the reality of the stoma becomes true. Hence, any psychological issues must be incorporated in the holistic nursing care plan. It is true to say that no two patients with newly formed stoma will react to their stoma formation in the same way. The two extracts below illustrate this:

. . . my initial concerns about my stoma related to its appearance, and the worries I had about intimacy . . . my fears were conveyed to my partner, resulting in less intimacy between us, it took longer than I expected to get used to this. (Female with ileostomy, aged 40, cited in White 1997)

. . . I live a full and normal life; I eat and drink what I want, I travel, work full-time, have relationships with men and try to live to the full. (Female ileostomy patient, aged 25, cited in White 1997)

When healthcare professionals are knowledgeable about body image and sexuality and secure with their own feelings they are more comfortable in dealing with these aspects of their work. The role of the nurse is to demonstrate knowledge regarding actual and potential problems associated with sexuality and an alteration in body image. In doing so, the nurse practitioner is assessing the meaning of alteration of both sexuality and body image for each individual patient and their family.

The nurse practitioner will need to acknowledge that different groups of patients will react in different ways to the creation of a stoma, for example, a patient with ulcerative colitis might accept a stoma as a positive concept in view of the constant diarrhoea with urgency plus the side-effects of its medical management whereas a patient with cancer may see the stoma as a negative concept as it becomes a constant reminder of the fact they once had cancer and possibly fear its return.

Effective communication and teamwork with other healthcare professionals is also essential in order for this group of patients and their relatives to receive the optimum level of care and information. For nurses to meet the needs of a patient who has a stoma it is important that they are aware of difficulties and understand the impact that a stoma may have on a person's health. Someone who has endured a chronic illness such as ulcerative colitis may well view their stoma in a positive manner whereas someone who has received a diagnosis of cancer resulting in stoma formation may view as negative, as the stoma brings about a constant reminder and in addition to this emotions experienced by pre-operative cancer patients are often concerned with the fear and uncertainty regarding the outcomes of treatment (Borwell 1997).

Excellent interpersonal skills such as listening, asking open-ended questions, using silence and summarising the discussion, will facilitate the sharing of information. This will help the patient make sense of and be able to accept the many changes that have occurred. During history taking the nurse should explore the patient's sexual activity prior to surgery and thus then can determine any pre-existing sexual concerns. Nurses should be confident of their own knowledge of sexuality and body image and be aware of their limitations and know when to refer the patient to another healthcare professional such as a counsellor or psychologist.

It is important that the patient receives information prior to stoma surgery but it is just as important that this information is appropriate for the patient's needs. The information should be sufficient enough to provide an outline of the proposed surgery and its potential complications. Involvement of other healthcare professionals such as the stoma care nurse can be invaluable at this point as they will be able to reinforce information previously given and supply written literature so that the patient can use it as a reference to prompt further questioning thus leading to a deeper understanding and ultimately easier adaptation.

The timing of the discussion with the patient is also important as immediately following surgery the patient is likely to be concerned with recovery and it is not until the basic needs have been addressed more complex issues of sexual concerns should be raised. Where these issues are discussed is also important. It is likely that the patient will want to discuss any issues in a private area and a busy surgical ward is not always appropriate. Discussions do not need to be planned and formal; patients are more likely to be open when they are in a relaxed private atmosphere, maybe while enjoying a bath.

It is well documented that patients who undergo stoma surgery experience similar grief and loss to those in the bereavement process (White 1998). These include loss of independence and confidence as their health fails and often loss of dignity. Some of these losses might be temporary but the loss of bowel or bladder function and the ability to function sexually can be permanent. The sense of loss and grief for someone with a stoma is often related to the loss of function, body parts and self-image. Additional losses may be associated with diagnosis, for example, where the disease may be perceived as life threatening. The severity of the grieving process will depend on past experiences and the value placed on the loss by the individual (Borwell 1997). This is considered to be a period of mourning. The role of the nurse is to encourage patients to talk about their experiences by using good communications skills as previously mentioned.

CONCLUSION

Stoma surgery involves a considerable degree of physical and psychological adjustment for all those who experience it. Excellent interpersonal skills, experience and knowledge of all aspects of stoma care are necessary for the nurse to distinguish between normal adjustment reactions and more psychological disturbances that may require in-depth therapeutic approaches.

Stoma surgery affects patients of all ages and adjustment to surgery must be made accordingly. Some stoma patients will return to a normal lifestyle with few problems while others may have more specific needs in order to adapt. In either case the nurse practitioner should be in a position to provide counselling and support before and after the surgery and to intervene so that the individual will be able to adapt to the alteration they are expressing in their body image and ultimately return to the lifestyle they previously enjoyed prior to the creation of the stoma (Salter 2002).

REFERENCES

Andersen, B.L. (1993) *Psychological Issues*. Williams and Wilkins, Baltimore.

Batchelor, D., Grahn, G., Oliver, G., Pritchard, P., Redmond, K. & Webb, P. (1991) *Cancer Care – Priorities for Nurses*. European Oncology Nursing Society, London.

Borwell, B. (1997) Psychological considerations of stoma care nursing. *Nursing Standard* **11**, 49–55.

Borwell, B. (1999) Sexuality and stoma care. In: P. Taylor, ed. *Stoma Care in the Community – A Clinical Resource for Practitioners.* NT Books, London.

Burnard, J. & Morrison, L. (1990) Body image and physical appearance. *Surgical Nurse* **3**, 4–8.

Cohen, A. (1991) Body image in a person with a stoma. *Journal of Enterostomal Therapy* **18**, 23–7.

Church, J. (1986) The current status of the Kock continent ileostomy. *Ostomy and Wound Management* Spring, 32–5.

Devlin, H., Plant, J. & Griffin, M. (1971) Aftermath of surgery for ano-rectal cancer. *British Medical Journal* **3**, 413–18.

Golis, A.M. (1996) Sexual issues for a person with an ostomy. *Journal of Wound, Ostomy and Continence Nursing* **23**, 33–7.

Kelman, G. & Minkler, P. (1989) An investigation of quality of life and self-esteem among individuals with ostomies. *Journal of Enterostomal Therapy* **16**, 4–11.

Klopp, A. (1990) Body image and self-esteem among individuals with stomas. *Journal of Enterostomal Therapy* **17**, 98–105.

Newell, R. (1991) Body image disturbance: cognitive behavioural formulation and intervention. *Journal of Advanced Nursing* **16**, 1400–5.

Nugent, K., Daniels, P., Stewart, B., Patankar, R. & Johnson, C.D. (1999) Quality of life in stoma patients. *Disease of the Colon and Rectum* **42**, 1569–74.

Pieper, B. & Mikols, C. (1996) Predischarge and postdischarge concerns of persons with an ostomy. *Journal of Wound, Ostomy and Continence Nursing* **23**, 105–9.

Price, B. (1990) *Body Image – Nursing Concepts and Care*. Prentice Hall, London.

Salter, M. (1997) *Altered Body Image: The Nurses Role*. 2nd edn. Baillière Tindall, London.

Salter, M. (2002) Sexual aspects of internal pouch surgery. In: J. Williams, ed. *The Essentials of Pouch Care Nursing*. Whurr Publishers, London.

Sprunk, E. & Alteneder, R.R. (2000) The impact of an ostomy on sexuality. *Clinical Journal of Oncology Nursing* **4**, 85–90.

Virgin-Elliston, T. (2003) Psychological considerations in stoma care. In: C. Elcoat, ed. *Stoma Care Nursing*. Hollister, Reading.

Wade, B. (1989) *A Stoma is for Life*. Scutari Press, London.

Wassner, A. (1992) The impact of mutilating surgery or trauma on body image. *International Nursing Review* **29**, 86–90.

Weerakoon, P. (2001) Sexuality and the patient with a stoma. *Sexuality and Disability* **19**, 121–9.

White, C. (1997) Psychological management of stoma-related concerns. *Nursing Standard* **12**, 35–8.

World Health Organization (1975) *Education and Treatment in Human Sexuality: The Training of Health Professionals*. WHO, Geneva.

Young-McCaughan, S. (1999) Invasive bladder cancer. In: C. Miaskowski & P. Buchel, eds. *Oncology Nursing: Assessment and Clinical Care*. Mosby, St. Louis.

Appendix
Useful Addresses

SUPPORT GROUPS

British Colostomy
   Association
15 Station Rd
Reading RG1 1LG
Tel: 0118 939 1537
Email: sue@bcass.org.uk
Website: www.bcass.org.uk

Ileostomy and Internal
   Pouch Association
PO Box 132
Scunthorpe DN15 9YW
Tel: 01724 720150
Email: ia@ileostomypouch.
   demon.co.uk
Website: www.
   ileostomypouch.demon.
   co.uk

National Association for
   Colitis and Crohn's
   Disease
PO Box 205
St Albans
Herts AL1 1AB
Tel: 01727 844296
Email: nacc@nacc.org.uk

Urostomy Association
Buckland
Beaumont Park
Danbury
Essex CM3 4DE
Tel: 01245 224294
Email: ua@centraloffice.fsnet.
   co.uk
Website: www.uagbi.org

Interstital Cystitis Support
   Group
76 High Street
Stony Stratford
Buckinghamshire MK11
   1AH
Website: www.
   interstitialcystitis.co.uk

Familial Adenomatous
   Polyposis (FAP) Support
   Group
Genetics Department,
   Birmingham Maternity
   Hospital
Edgbaston, Birmingham
West Midlands, B13 9TB
Tel: 0121 6272632
Website: www.clinical-
   genetics@virgin.net

CANCER-RELATED SUPPORT AGENCIES

BACUP
3 Bath Place
London EC2A 3JR
Tel: 0207 696 9003
Website: www.cancerbacup.
　org.uk

Cancerlink
11–21 Northdown Street
London N1 9BN
Tel: 0207 833 2818
Email:
　cancerlink@cancerlink.org
Website: www.cancerlink.org

Colon Cancer Concern
4 Rickett Street
London SW6 1RU
Infoline: 08708 506050
Email:
　admin@coloncancer.org.uk
Website:
　www.coloncancer.org.uk

Cancer Research UK
Tel: 020 7242 0200
Website: www.
　cancerresearchuk.org

Cancer Care Society
11 The Cornmarket
Romsey
Hampshire SO51 8GB
Tel: 01794 830300
Website: www.cancercaresoc.
　demon.co.uk

Beating Bowel Cancer
PO Box 360
Twickenham TW1 1UN
Tel: 020 8892 5256
Email:
　info@beatingbowelcancer.
　org

Macmillan Cancer Relief
89 Albert Embankment
London SE1 7UQ
Tel: 0845 601 601
　(information line)
Website:
　www.macmillan.org.uk

AGENCIES SUPPORTING SEXUAL/RELATIONSHIP PROBLEMS

Relate
Herbert Gray College
Little Church Street
Rugby CV21 3AP

SPOD (Sexual problems of
the disabled)
286 Camden Street
London N7 0BJ

Gay Ostomists Association
Tel: 0151 726 9019
Email:
gay.ostomates@virgin.net
Website:
www.welcome.to/gay.
ostomates

Impotence Information
Centre
PO Box 1130
London W3 9BB

British Association for
Counselling (BAC)
1 Regents Place
Rugby CV21 2PJ
Tel: 01788 578328

British Association of Sexual
and Marital Therapy
PO Box 62
Sheffield S10 3TS

CLOTHING
SASH Stoma Support and
Hernia Belt
Woodhouse,
Woodside Road
Hockley
Essex SS5 4RU
Website:
www.sashstomabelts.com

Fittleworth Medical Limited
(support garments)
Unit L Rudford Industrial
Estate
Ford, Arundel
West Sussex BN1 0BD
Tel: 01903 732056

Salts (support garments)
Salt and Son Ltd
Lord Street
Birmingham B7 4DS
Tel: 0121 359 5123

PROFESSIONAL NURSING
RCN Stoma Care and
Gastroenterology Forum
RCN Cardiff
Tel: 01222 553411

English National Board for
Nursing, Midwifery and
Health Visiting
Victory House
170 Tottenham Court Road
London W1P 0HA

Glossary

Acute	Sudden onset of symptoms.
Adhesion	Internal scar tissue following abdominal or pelvic surgery.
Alimentary tract	Digestive tube from the mouth to the anus.
Anal sphincter	Opening and closing muscles of the anus, both involuntary and voluntary muscles.
Anastomosis	Surgical joining of two ends of bowel, may be stapled or hand sewn.
Anorectum	The last 12 cm (5 inches) of bowel.
Anus	The outlet of the rectum lying in the fold between the buttocks, approximately 5 cm (2 inches) long.
Appliance	The bag or pouch worn over a stoma.
Bladder cancer	Rarely occurs under the age of 50 but is thought to be linked with environmental factors such as dyes and industrial chemicals. Often treated by local excision (transurethral resection) but larger, more invasive tumours will necessitate bladder excision.
Bladder exstrophy	A condition in which the anterior wall of the bladder, the roof of the urethra and parts of the abdominal wall are missing. In some cases reconstruction of the bladder is possible but in many cases urinary diversion or ileal conduit is necessary.

Caecum	The first part of the large bowel which accepts liquid contents from the ileum.
Cloacal exstrophy	A condition in which the bladder, ureters and bowel are exposed. Often associated with other congenital abnormalities. A urinary and faecal stoma will be required.
Colectomy	The surgical removal of all or part of the large bowel.
Colitis	Inflammation of the mucosa of the colon. Causes bloody diarrhoea and urgency. Many patients are managed medically on steroids and anti-inflammatory drugs but in some the condition cannot be controlled and surgical removal of the colon is required.
Colon	The large bowel from ileum to rectum, approximately 1.5 m (60 inches) long.
Colon cancer	Colorectal cancer is the second biggest cancer killer in the UK and most commonly occurs in those over 65.
Colostomy	An opening with a 'bag' allowing semi-solid bowel contents to pass from the colon to the exterior. Part of the colon is brought out of the abdomen creating a stoma.
Constipation	Infrequent or difficulty in the passage of bowel motion (stool, faeces).
Crohn's disease	An inflammatory bowel disease which can affect any part of the gastrointestinal tract from the mouth to the anus. Symptoms are similar to ulcerative colitis but abdominal pain is much more pronounced. Surgical intervention is limited to treating the complications of Crohn's disease such

as strictures and entero-cutaneous fistulae.

Cystectomy Surgical removal of all or a part of the bladder.

Distal Further down the bowel towards the anus.

Diverticular disease Pockets in the wall of the large bowel which may become inflamed and infected with stagnant faeces.

Familial adenomatous polyposis A condition in which multiple polyps are found throughout the gastrointestinal tract. This is inherited as an autosomal dominant trait.

Flange The piece that is bonded to the skin barrier. It provides a secure connection for the pouch.

Flatulence Excessive gas in the intestines.

Heredity The transmission of characteristics from parent to child.

Hirschsprung's disease An ultra-small area of the colon or anorectum without the normal nerve supply, so normal function is not possible.

Ileal conduit See urostomy.

Ileo-anal pouch A pouch fashioned from the ileum which is then anastomosed to the anus for the restoration of normal continence.

Ileostomy An opening with a bag to collect liquid contents from the small bowel, used when the colon and anorectum are diseased.

Ileum The last part of the small bowel, from 4.5 m (15 feet) to 9.5 m (31 feet) long.

Incontinence Involuntary loss of urine or faeces or both.

Irradiation damage The bowel is sensitive to irradiation. Radiation given to treat gynaecological or bladder cancers may damage the bowel resulting in abdominal pain and bloody diarrhoea. Strictures can occur and surgical excision of the damaged segment of bowel may be required.

Ischaemia Inadequate flow of blood caused by constriction or blockage.

Jejunum The part of the small bowel between the duodenum (not the stomach) and ileum (near the large bowel); about 2.5 m (8 feet) long.

Kock pouch An internal pouch which is constructed using the small bowel. A valve is created at the point where the pouch meets the abdominal wall. The valve then gives the patient control over the emptying of the bowel.

Laparotomy Surgical incision into the abdominal cavity.

Malabsorption Inability to fully absorb nutrients in the small intestine.

Mitrofanoff pouch This pouch may be formed using the bladder or bowel or both. The pouch is joined to the skin via a tunnel which is constructed using bowel tissue. The pouch can be emptied of urine by using a catheter.

Motility This is the movement of food and chemicals through the alimentary tract.

Mucous A white slimy lubricant produced by the large bowel as a mechanism to lubricate the bowel.

Mucous fistula	This is formed from the distal end of divided bowel which is brought to the surface. It no longer functions for the disposal of waste, however, it will continue to secrete mucous.
Nasogastric tube	Tube inserted through the nose and down into the stomach.
Necrosis	Dead tissue.
Oedema	Accumulation (build up) of excessive amounts of fluid in the tissues resulting in swelling.
Oesophagus	The muscular tube from the mouth to the stomach approximately 23 cm (9 inches) long.
One-piece appliance	This is where the wafer is bonded to the pouch.
Ostomist	A person who undergoes stoma formation.
Perforation	An abnormal opening (hole) in the bowel wall which causes the contents to spill into the normally sterile abdominal cavity.
Pelvic floor muscles	The complex group of supporting, and opening and closing muscles, involved in urinary, sexual and anorectal function.
Perineum	This is the superficial tissue from the vulva to anus in the female and from the scrotum to anus in male.
Peristalsis	Contraction of the muscular walls of the alimentary tract necessary to push food and gases along.
Peritoneum	Membrane lining the inside of the abdominal activity.
Peritonitis	Inflammation of the peritoneum.

Polyps	Benign, pre-malignant or malignant growths commonly found in the colon and rectum.
Proctocolectomy	Removal of rectum and colon.
Proximal	Further up the bowel towards the mouth.
Rectal cancer	Cancer of the terminal part of the large intestine.
Rectum	The large intestine, above the anus (the back passage).
Reflux	Backward flow of liquid.
Retraction	Pulling back.
Sigmoid colon	An S-shaped part of the descending colon leading to the rectum. It can act as a 'brake' on the movement of faeces to the rectum.
Suppository	A rectal medication shaped like a pellet, inserted into the rectum.
Stenosis	Narrowing.
Stoma	Part of the bowel visible on the surface of the abdomen after surgery.
Stomal rod (bridge)	A plastic rod that keeps the loop of bowel in place and prevents it from retracting into the abdomen. The rod can be removed 7–10 days after surgery.
Stricture	The narrowing of a portion of the bowel.
Terminal ileum	The last part of the ileum joining the caecum via the ileocaecal value.
Tumour	An abnormal growth which may be benign (non-cancerous) or malignant (cancer).
Two-piece appliance	A two piece consists of a wafer which is attached to the skin. The wafer will

	usually have a flange attached to allow for a secure connection of the bag.
Ulcerative colitis	Ulceration and inflammation of the large bowel.
Urethra	This is the opening from the bladder, allowing urine to pass to the exterior.
Urostomy	Surgical creation of an external opening into the ureter, which usually involves bringing the ureter to the skin surface so that urine can drain into an appliance.
Volvulus	A sigmoid volvulus occurs when the sigmoid colon becomes twisted on its blood supply causing obstruction. Surgery is required to prevent bowel ischaemia.

Index

Page numbers in **bold** indicate tables